Management of Prostate Diseases

Second Edition

Robert E. Weiss, MD

Assistant Professor of Urology
Department of Surgery
UMDNJ Robert Wood Johnson Medical Center
New Brunswick, NJ

William R. Fair, MD

Professor and Chief
Urology Service
Department of Surgery
Memorial Sloan-Kettering Cancer Center
New York, NY

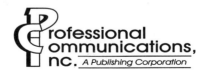

Professional
Communications,
Inc. *A Publishing Corporation*

Published by:
Professional Communications, Inc.

For orders only, please call:
1-800-337-9838

ISBN: 1-884735-24-X

Printed in the United States of America

ACKNOWLEDGMENT

The authors wish to acknowledge Jean Fitzpatrick for her assistance in preparing the manuscript for this updated edition.

TABLE OF CONTENTS

TABLES

FIGURES

Introduction

The last few years have seen several advances in the diagnosis and management of prostate disease, including:

- Prostate-specific antigen (PSA) screening for prostate cancer
- 5α-reductase inhibitor and long-acting α_1-adrenergic-receptor-antagonist drugs for benign prostatic hyperplasia
- A promising new prostate-specific α_{1A} subtype adrenoceptor antagonist
- Achievement of complete androgen source ablation with a combination of a luteinizing hormone-releasing hormone (LHRH) agonist and a nonsteroidal antiandrogen agent
- Transurethral laser prostatectomy
- Transurethral microwave thermotherapy
- Transperineal cryosurgery.

With the increase in older patients entering today's diverse medical care systems, primary-care physicians are seeing more prostate disease, which in its several manifestations can require an increasingly sophisticated understanding of etiologies, differential diagnoses, and therapeutic interventions.

Designed to provide primary-care physicians with a review of the basics of prostatic disease, as well as updated guidelines for initial evaluation and consultation, this second edition of the handbook on *Management of Prostate Diseases* outlines what we now know about the etiology, diagnosis, and treatment of infection, hypertrophic changes, and cancer of the prostate.

Prostatitis, one of the most common infections in men, affects those of all ages, ranging from the young, sexually active to the debilitated, elderly patient with urinary retention. Often a diagnostic challenge, prostatitis is classified into four types:

- Acute bacterial
- Chronic bacterial
- Nonbacterial
- Prostatodynia.

Benign prostatic hyperplasia (BPH) is primarily a condition of older men. Ten years ago, approximately 400,000 men underwent surgery annually for BPH. More recently, the introduction of pharmaceutical therapy has made this surgery unnecessary in most cases. Newer modalities such as laser ablation and microwave hyperthermia promise an even greater range of minimally invasive interventions.

Prostate cancer, which represents 20% of all newly diagnosed neoplasms in American men, is being diagnosed and treated at an earlier stage than ever before through the use of serum PSA testing and rectal sonography-guided biopsy.

Finally, we present several case histories describing typical presentations of prostatic disease with relevant therapeutic interventions.

We hope this handbook will serve as a guide for primary-care physicians and health-care workers in the evaluation, initial treatment, and appropriate referral of patients. In short, we have designed the handbook to be the basis of a working relationship between the primary-care physician and the urologist for the benefit of all patients with prostatic disease.

PART 1

THE PROSTATE

1

Anatomy and Anatomical Relationships of the Prostate

The walnut-sized, 20 g prostate is a fibromuscular and glandular organ that encircles the urethra at the bladder neck. Enlargement or inflammation and swelling of the prostate can obstruct the urethra. The seminal vesicles converge toward the base of the prostate gland where each joins with the corresponding vas deferens to form the ejaculatory ducts. The ejaculatory ducts open into the prostatic urethra at the verumontanum (Figure 1.1). During ejaculation, the seminal fluid mixes with sperm in the prostate. The bladder neck closes to prevent retrograde ejaculation, and the ejaculate is propelled forward through the penis.

Components of the prostate include:
- Outer, thin, firm fibrous capsule
- Dense layer of muscular tissue
- Dense layer of circular fibers around urethra
- Excretory ducts and prostatic ducts
- Columnar epithelium lining the excretory ducts.

Blood vessels supplying and lymphatics draining the prostate include (Figure 1.2):
- Arteries
  - Inferior vesical
  - Internal pudendal
  - Middle rectal (hemorrhoidal)
- Veins
  - Periprostatic plexus, drains into deep dorsal vein
  - Internal iliacs
- Lymphatic drainage
  - Internal iliac

FIGURE 1.1 — THE PROSTATE AND SURROUNDING ORGANS

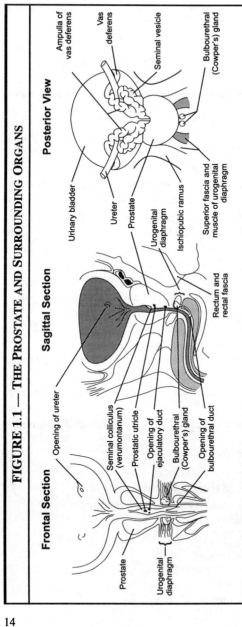

The anatomical relationships of the prostate gland, which contribute approximately 5% to 15% of semen, are shown here in frontal and sagittal section and posterior view.

FIGURE 1.2 — SCHEMATICS OF PROSTATE ARTERIAL CIRCULATION AND LYMPHATIC SYSTEM

Arterial Circulation

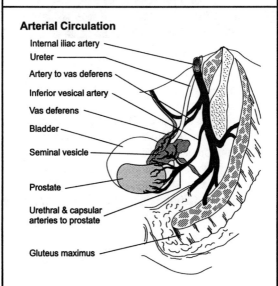

Internal iliac artery
Ureter
Artery to vas deferens
Inferior vesical artery
Vas deferens
Bladder
Seminal vesicle
Prostate
Urethral & capsular arteries to prostate
Gluteus maximus

Lymphatic System

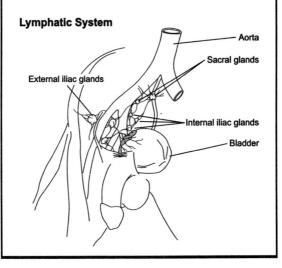

Aorta
Sacral glands
External iliac glands
Internal iliac glands
Bladder

15

- Sacral
- External iliac nodes.

Normal Prostatic Resistance to Infection

The prostate has several mechanisms of resistance to infection, including:

- Its secretory function, which opposes ascending infection
- Prostatic antibacterial factor, free zinc, which is bactericidal to most organisms that cause common genitourinary tract infections
- Activity of spermatozoa against gram-positive bacteria
- Local IgG/IgA response specific to infecting pathogens.

PART 2

PROSTATITIS

2

Prostatitis: Classification and Presentation

Prostatitis can range from an acute bacterial infection, which may be associated with potentially life-threatening sepsis, to chronic vague discomfort or persistent pain with negative microscopic examination and culture. The syndromes have been classified into four categories according to clinical findings:

- Acute bacterial prostatitis
- Chronic bacterial prostatitis
- Nonbacterial prostatitis
- Prostatodynia (PD).

Prostatitis is, therefore, not a single disease with one etiology, but rather several different diseases with different clinical features (Table 2.1).

Acute Bacterial Prostatitis

Most often an infection of young men, acute bacterial prostatitis (ABP) is usually caused by the ascent of an infecting organism up the urethra and reflux of infected urine into the prostatic ducts. Lymphatic and hematogenous routes are also possible but much less common. It is also associated with Foley catheterization and cystoscopy.

Acute bacterial prostatitis is characterized by:

- Rapid onset
- Fever
- Chills
- Suprapubic, flank, and perineal pain
- Dysuria
- Urinary frequency and urgency

19

TABLE 2.1 — CLINICAL FEATURES OF COMMON PROSTATITIS SYNDROMES

Syndrome	History of Confirmed UTI	Prostate Abnormal on Rectal Exam	Excessive WBCs in EPS	Positive Culture of EPS	Common Causative Agents	Response to Antimicrobial Treatment	Impaired Urinary Flow Rate
Acute bacterial prostatitis	Yes	Yes	Yes	Yes	Coliform bacteria	Yes	Yes
Chronic bacterial prostatitis	Yes	±	Yes	Yes	Coliform bacteria	Yes	±
Nonbacterial prostatitis	No	±	Yes	No	None ? *Chlamydia* ? *Ureaplasma*	Usually no	±
Prostatodynia	No	No	No	No	None	No	Yes

Abbreviations: UTI, urinary tract infection; WBCs, white blood cells; EPS, expressed prostatic secretions.

Reprinted from Meares EM Jr. Prostatitis and related disorders. In: Walsh PC, Retik AB, Stamey TA, eds. *Campbell's Urology*. Volume 1. Philadelphia, Pa: WB Saunders Co; 1992:807-822.

- Tense, boggy, acutely tender prostate on rectal examination (should be gentle to prevent bacteremia).

Prostate massage is contraindicated; however, the etiologic agent is usually evident on urine gram stain and culture. The most common causative organisms are gram-negative enteric bacteria, similar to those found in urinary tract infections (UTIs):
- *Escherichia coli*
- Proteus
- Klebsiella
- Enterobacteria
- Pseudomonas
- Serratia.

Enterococcus has also been identified in prostatitis but less commonly.

Chronic Bacterial Prostatitis

Although chronic bacterial prostatitis (CBP) can evolve from the acute disease, many patients have no history of acute infection. Clinical manifestations are variable. Some patients may be asymptomatic but most have varying degrees of irritative voiding symptoms. Many report a history of UTIs. Presentation usually includes:
- Nocturia, dysuria, urinary frequency
- Perineal pain without fever or chills
- Low back pain
- Mildly to exquisitely tender prostate
- Microscopic evidence of inflammation
- Positive culture.

Sequential urine/expressed prostatic secretion (EPS) sampling should be done, with culture of urethral, bladder, and prostatic secretions.

Nonbacterial Prostatitis

The most common of the prostatitis syndromes, nonbacterial prostatitis (NBP), is an inflammatory disorder of unknown cause. A number of etiologies have been suggested, however:

- Some investigators believe it may be an autoimmune disease.
- Recent work suggests that both NBP and PD may be secondary to interstitial cystitis.
- The prostatic fluid of men with NBP has been reported to show weak but definite mean antigen-specific antibody elevations in response to mixes of *Escherichia coli* serogroups and of other enteric, gram-negative bacteria commonly responsible for UTIs.

Presenting symptoms of nonbacterial prostatitis are similar to those of CBP. Expressed prostatic secretions show increased leukocytes and lipid-laden macrophages but the diagnosis is made primarily by exclusion. Patients will have:

- A negative culture
- No history of UTI
- No history of prostatitis.

Prostatodynia

A noninflammatory disorder that affects young and middle-aged men, PD represents one of the more perplexing prostate problems. Patients usually present with:

- Suprapubic, perineal, and pelvic pain
- Dysuria
- Urinary frequency.

Rectal examination is usually normal, cultures are negative, and EPS contain no leukocytes or lipid-laden macrophages. Examination of EPS is crucial to distinguish PD from the prostatitis syndromes. Cystoscopic and urodynamic testing for possible neurologic or anatomical causes has resulted in suggestions that PD may be the result of:

- Chronic tension in the muscles of the pelvic floor
- A history of hemorrhoids/constipation
- Neuromuscular dysfunction (lack of external sphincter relaxation, bladder neck spasm).

Investigators have also postulated etiologic roles for:

- Emotional instability
- Stress (resulting in diminished host immunity)
- Coagulase-negative Staphylococcus species, which have antiphagocytic, antichemotactic, and lymphocyte antiproliferative properties
- Intrapelvic venous congestion
- Interstitial cystitis.

3 Diagnosis

Acute bacterial prostatitis (ABP) can usually be diagnosed on the basis of typical symptoms and signs, pyuria and bacteriuria. However, symptoms of chronic bacterial and nonbacterial prostatitis, as well as those of prostatodynia overlap. Thus, in addition to a detailed patient history and physical examination, patients should be evaluated with sequential urine/expressed prostatic secretion (EPS) sampling.

History

In addition to current signs and symptoms, history should include information regarding:
- Past prostatic problems or urinary tract infections (UTIs)
- Recent urethral instrumentation and/or rectal examination
- Immunosuppressive disease or therapy.

Physical Examination

Patients presenting with the signs and symptoms of prostatic disease should undergo a comprehensive differential examination for:
- Fever, a sign of acute disease with possible bacteremia, rules out other forms of prostatitis and prostatodynia
- Prostate inflammation (fluctuance suggests presence of an abscess)
- Flank pain, which may be indicative of
  - Renal colic (pain intermittent)
  - Pyelonephritis (pain dull, continuous)

- Bladder distention (urinary retention often occurs with acute bacterial prostatitis)
- Cystitis, due to UTI
- Epididymitis, often a site of infection in UTI (Figure 3.1)
- Urethritis, usually associated with dysuria (whitish discharge on urethral massage)
- Rectal/perianal fissures, fistula, abscess
- Hemorrhoids.

Microscopic Examination

Differentiation of the three nonacute prostatic syndromes—chronic bacterial prostatitis, nonbacterial prostatitis, and prostatodynia—is accomplished by microscopic examination of the patient's urine and prostatic secretions by sequential urine and EPS sampling (in acute disease, EPS are excluded since prostatic massage is contraindicated) (Table 3.1).

The urine/EPS samples are divided into four categories (Figure 3.2):
- **Voided Bladder 1** (VB_1), the initial 5 to 10 mL of urine voided, for identification of urethral bacteria. Then patient should void approximately 150 cc to clear urethra.
- **Voided Bladder 2** (VB_2), midstream specimen for identification of bladder bacteria, after which patient should interrupt voiding.
- **EPS**: With patient in knee/chest position, prostate is gently massaged from base to apex to empty prostatic ducts (Figure 3.3). Perineal massage will bring secretions to penile meatus.
- **Voided Bladder 3** (VB_3), first 10 mL collected immediately after prostatic massage.

Urine specimens are sent for urinalysis, and both urine and EPS samples, for culture and sensitivity testing (C&S). For a diagnosis of CBP, comparison of

3

FIGURE 3.1 — PROGRESSION OF PROSTATE INFECTION

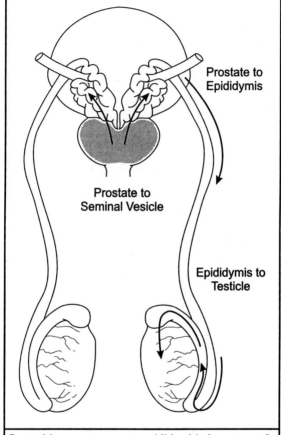

Prostate to Epididymis

Prostate to Seminal Vesicle

Epididymis to Testicle

Prostatitis can progress to epididymitis by retrograde spread of bacteria.

the bacteria counts of all three cultures must clearly show excessive bacteria in the semen.

Localization of the site of inflammation to urethra or prostate requires comparison of the micro-

TABLE 3.1 — MICROSCOPIC EXAMINATION OF SEQUENTIAL URINE SAMPLING

Urine Sample	Results of Microscopic Examination	Possible Diagnosis
Centrifuged VB_2	Bacteria visible; bacteria > 5 leukocytes/HPF (because of bacturia)	Acute or chronic prostatitis; acute or chronic cystitis
	Bacteria not visible	Nonbacterial prostatitis (unremarkable) or prostadynia (unremarkable)
VB_1	Many leukocytes (should be > 5X leukocytes in VB_2)	Urethritis/cystitis
EPS	Many leukocytes > 10 leukocytes/HPF; lipid-laden macrophages; alteration of prostatic fluid LDH 5:1 ratio	Indicative of inflammation

Abbreviations: VB, voided bladder; HPF, high power field; LDH, lactate dehydrogenase.

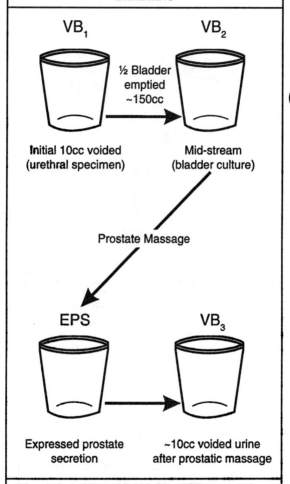

FIGURE 3.2 — SEQUENTIAL URINE/EPS SAMPLING

VB_1 VB_2

½ Bladder emptied ~150cc

Initial 10cc voided (urethral specimen)

Mid-stream (bladder culture)

Prostate Massage

EPS VB_3

Expressed prostate secretion

~10cc voided urine after prostatic massage

Abbreviations: VB, voided bladder; EPS, expressed prostatic secretion.

Culture of specimens collected as illustrated here help to localize pathogenic bacteria to urethra, bladder, or prostate.

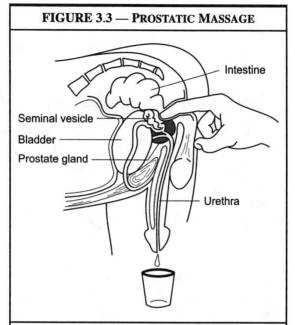

FIGURE 3.3 — PROSTATIC MASSAGE

Collection of prostatic secretions is achieved by prostatic massage, for which the patient assumes the knee-chest position and prostate acini are emptied by massaging from base to apex with the gloved finger.

scopic appearance of the EPS to smears of the spun sediment of VB_1 and VB_2:

- If VB_2 (bladder specimen) is sterile, prostate colonization or infection is indicated by a much higher (ten-fold) bacterial count obtained from the EPS and VB_3 specimens.
- Conversely, urethral infection is indicated by a higher count from the VB_1 culture.

A high VB_2 count indicates bladder colonization and requires an antimicrobial agent active in urine but not in tissues (penicillin G).

FIGURE 3.4 — LOCALIZING THE INFECTION

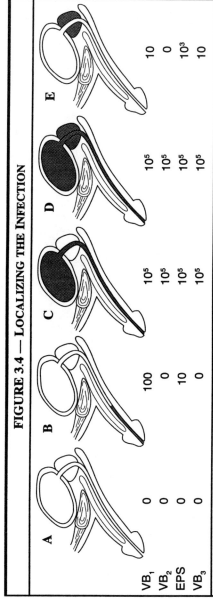

	A	B	C	D	E
VB_1	0	100	10^5	10^5	10
VB_2	0	0	10^5	10^5	0
EPS	0	10	10^5	10^5	10^3
VB_3	0	0	10^5	10^5	10

Abbreviations: VB, voided bladder; EPS, expressed prostatic secretion.

Culture results from sequentially collected urethral urine, bladder urine, prostatic expressate, and post-prostatic massage urine can localize the infection. A = negative cultures; no infection. B = VB_1, the urethral specimen is positive, suggesting urethritis. C = bacteriuria. D = bacteriuria + prostatitis. E = prostatitis alone.

31

Results of urine/EPS sampling with possible diagnosis are seen in Table 3.1 and Figure 3.4.

4 Treatment

Because prostatitis occurs in several distinct forms or syndromes, each of which has separate causes, clinical features, and sequelae, clinical management requires both specific diagnosis and therapeutic strategy. For example, in acute bacterial infection, the intense, diffuse inflammatory reaction enhances the passage of antibacterial agents, whether acidic or alkaline, from plasma into the prostatic secretory system. In the chronic bacterial syndrome, however, the prostate fluid's increased alkalinity as well as the less marked inflammatory response favors the diffusion of acidic antimicrobial agents from plasma across prostatic epithelium into the fluid.

Other antimicrobial characteristics specific to permeation of chronic bacterial prostatitis' (CBP) nonacutely inflamed lipid membrane include:
- High lipid solubility
- Minimal binding to plasma proteins
- Activity against gram-negative bacteria.

Eradication of prostatic foci of infection is often difficult because:
- Many antimicrobial agents do not diffuse well across the prostatic epithelium into prostatic fluid.
- Calculi, the result of precipitation of stones from refluxed urine or of inspissation and calcification of prostatic secretions, can block drainage of portions of the gland or act as foreign bodies.
- An enlarged or inflamed prostate can cause bladder outlet obstruction resulting in pools of stagnant, difficult-to-sterilize urine in the bladder.

Acute Bacterial Prostatitis

The etiologic agent in acute bacterial prostatitis (ABP), which can usually be identified on urine gram stain and culture, is generally a common gram-negative urinary tract pathogen (*Escherichia Coli* or Klebsiella). The patient should be started on either:

- Ciprofloxacin, 500 mg, bid for 10 days
  OR
- Trimethoprim, 80 mg, and sulfamethoxazole, 400 mg (TMP-SMX), 2 tablets, bid for 10 days.

In catheter-associated infections, a broader spectrum of etiologic agents is seen, including hospital-acquired gram-negative rods and enterococci. Such infections should be treated with an aminoglycoside, a fluoroquinolone, or a third-generation cephalosporin until the organism has been isolated and susceptibilities determined.

Hospitalization and intravenous antimicrobials are necessary for patients who are febrile with symptoms of systemic infection. Initial therapy should be:

- Ampicillin, 1 g, q6hrs; and gentamicin, 80 mg, q8hrs or longer depending on renal function
- Antimicrobial agents to be adjusted on return of culture results.

Intravenous therapy may also be advisable for those who:

- Are debilitated by age
- Appear toxic
- Have a concomitant illness
- Are immunocompromised.

Acute urinary retention should be managed by percutaneous placement of a suprapubic catheter by a urologist. Transurethral catheters are poorly tolerated and may lead to complications.

34

Chronic Bacterial Prostatitis

Antibacterial therapy should be initiated as soon as positive culture results are received. Antimicrobials promptly relieve the symptoms of CBP but apparently are less effective in removing the focus of infection. Thus patients return frequently with renewed discomfort and recurrent infection. The following antimicrobial regimens, listed in order of clinical efficacy, should be given for 10 to 14 days:

- TMP-SMX, 2 tablets, bid
- Ciprofloxacin, 500 mg, bid
- Carbenicillin, 2 tablets, qid
- Tetracycline, 250 to 500 mg, qid (for 10 days)
- Doxycycline, 100 mg, bid
- Erythromycin, 250 to 500 mg, qid.

Long-term treatment (4 to 12 months) has been attempted, with some improvement in symptoms. Some investigators have tried direct injection of antimicrobial agents into the prostate without significant success. Others have suggested low-dose suppressive antibacterial therapy. Treatment is often dependent on the patient's individual response.

Transurethral resection of the prostate (TURP, see Chapter 7) should be considered a last resort. TURP is not usually effective unless CBP is caused by:

- Prostatic calculi
- Prostatic duct obstruction as a result of prostatic abscess.

Prostatic Abscess

Abscess may be the result of acute prostatitis and often occurs in immunocompromised patients, such as those with:

- Diabetes mellitus

- Human immunodeficiency virus (HIV) infection
- Long-term, indwelling Foley catheter.

Treatment of prostatic abscess should include:
- Intravenous ampicillin, 1 g, q6hrs; and gentamicin, 80 mg, q8hrs, or longer depending on renal function (Antimicrobial agents may be adjusted on return of culture results.)
- Prompt incision and drainage by a urologist.

Prostatitis and Infertility

Although acute prostatitis may decrease sperm motility, resolution of the infection should return fertility to normal. Many clinicians believe that the increased alkalinity of the prostatic fluid in chronic bacterial disease has adverse effects on spermatozoa, with resultant subfertility. Whether chronic prostatitis can lead to chronic subfertility is still controversial, however. Most studies have shown little improvement in fertility rates in men with CBP despite antimicrobial therapy.

Nonbacterial Prostatitis

Because its etiology is unknown, effective treatment of nonbacterial prostatitis (NBP) is difficult to achieve. Although cultures generally exclude the usual bacterial pathogens, a trial of tetracycline, doxycycline, or erythromycin (see CBP dosages) may be a reasonable precaution. Then the following measures may be helpful:
- Patient reassurance
- Encouragement of exercise and normal sexual activity
- Avoidance of caffeine, ethyl alcohol, spicy foods

- Warm sitz baths
- Anti-inflammatory agents, such as:
  - Ibuprofen, 400 mg, qid or with meals, as needed
  - Indomethacin, 25 to 50 mg, tid with meals, as needed
- An anticholinergic agent, such as oxybutynin chloride, 5 mg, at bedtime for voiding urgency.

Prostatodynia

Treatment of prostatodynia (PD) usually consists of an initial 10- to 14-day course of antibiotics, such as:
- TMP-SMX, 2 tablets, bid
  OR
- Tetracycline, 250 to 500 mg, qid.

Patients generally do not respond to antimicrobial therapy so no further trials are warranted. Subsequent treatment should include:
- Reassurance that no infection or malignancy is present
- Warm sitz baths
- An α_1-adrenergic blocking agent to relax the urinary sphincter
  - Terazosin (Hytrin), 1 mg, qd; may increase to 5 mg qd, but must monitor blood pressure (bp)
  - Doxazosin mesylate (Cardura), 1 mg, qd; may increase to 2 or 4 mg, qd, but must monitor bp
- Diazepam, 2 mg, tid, as needed, for tension myalgia of the pelvic floor
- Biofeedback.

Symptoms of PD are usually found in men with "type A" personalities in high stress situations. Therefore, lifestyle modification may represent the only effective cure.

PART 3

BENIGN PROSTATIC HYPERPLASIA

5

Description, Presentation of Benign Prostatic Hyperplasia

The prostate gland begins increasing in size at puberty and reaches adult size of about 20 g by age 20. It remains stable in size for about 25 years, with a second growth spurt beginning during the fifth decade in the majority of men. Thus, benign prostatic hyperplasia (BPH) affects men over the age of 45 and increases in frequency with age (Figure 5.1). Nearly 25% of men 60 to 69 years of age have enlarged prostates, and by the eighth decade more than 90% have prostatic hyperplasia at autopsy.

Benign prostatic hyperplasia is a heterogeneous disorder caused by hormonal factors, growth factors, stromal-epithelial interactions, and aging. A histological diagnosis, BPH frequently progresses to benign prostatic enlargement (BPE), benign prostatic obstruction (BPO), and lower urinary tract symptoms (LUTS).

The amount of hyperplasia as well as degree of prostatic enlargement required to cause symptoms varies among patients. However, classical LUTS include:

- Hesitancy
- Incomplete emptying of bladder
- Straining to void
- Nocturia
- Poor stream.

Pathophysiology

Recent studies of the pharmacologic treatment of BPH have resulted in the recognition that the condi-

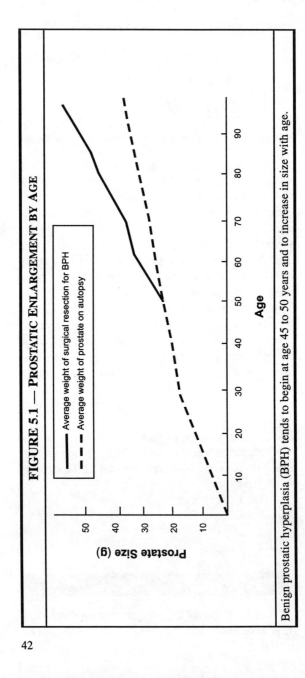

FIGURE 5.1 — PROSTATIC ENLARGEMENT BY AGE

Average weight of surgical resection for BPH
Average weight of prostate on autopsy

Prostate Size (g)

Age

Benign prostatic hyperplasia (BPH) tends to begin at age 45 to 50 years and to increase in size with age.

42

tion is not a single entity in which an enlarged gland causes symptoms. Men with small glands may also be symptomatic.

Prostatic hyperplasia arises as spherical masses of epithelial and stromal elements from the glands lining the proximal prostatic urethra (Figure 5.2). As the masses enlarge, they form lobes of varying configuration and, in turn varying degrees of mechanical obstruction. For example, obstruction may occur with relatively little prostatic enlargement, given selective hyperplasia of the middle lobe, which is strategically placed to encroach on the bladder neck (Figure 5.3).

The ratio of epithelium to smooth muscle in the prostate can vary substantially among individual men, from 1:3 to 4:1. In general, however, larger prostates contain more androgen-dependent epithelial elements than smaller glands, which contain a higher proportion of smooth muscle. In either case, the outcome of BPH may be urethral obstruction, induced mechanically by epithelial overgrowth and dynamically by smooth muscle contraction, or by a combination of both.

Staged Bladder Response

The bladder reacts to obstruction in stages, with **Stage I** characterized by bladder irritability, resulting in:
- Urinary frequency
- Nocturia.

Stage II represents compensatory changes:
- Thickened detrusor musculature
- Urinary hesitancy
- Decreased force of urinary stream
- High pressure voiding to evacuate urine.

FIGURE 5.2 — ANATOMY OF PROSTATIC HYPERPLASIA

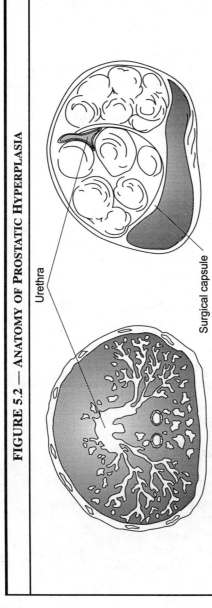

Urethra

Surgical capsule

Normal and hyperplastic prostates are compared here in cross section. Note the severe narrowing of the prostatic urethra as well as the surgical capsule formed by the hyperplastic masses compressing the prostate's outer zone.

Adapted from Walsh PC. Benign prostatic hyperplasia. In: Walsh PC, Retik AB, Stamey TA, eds. *Campbell's Urology.* Volume 1. Philadelphia, Pa: WB Saunders Co; 1992:1011.

FIGURE 5.3 — SITES OF PROSTATIC HYPERPLASIA

Isolated Middle
Lobe Enlargement

Isolated Lateral
Lobe Enlargement

Lateral and Middle
Lobe Enlargement

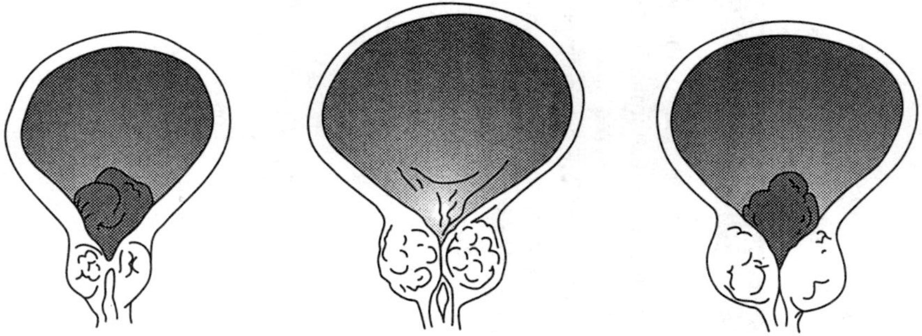

"Lobes" of hyperplastic prostatic tissue are seen obstructing the prostatic urethra. An isolated middle-lobe may occur in a relatively small prostate, whereas lateral and middle lobes of hyperplasia result in an obviously enlarged organ.

Adapted from Walsh PC. Benign prostatic hyperplasia. In: Walsh PC, Retik AB, Stamey TA, eds. *Campbell's Urology*. Volume 1. Philadelphia, Pa: WB Saunders Co; 1992:1013.

Stage III, decompensation:
- Slowing of urine stream to a dribble
- Enlargement of the bladder
- Loss of bladder tone (floppy bladder)
- Bladder sensation loss (no sense of fullness)
- Urinary stasis with:
  - Pressure backup
  - Dilated ureters and hydronephrosis
  - Azotemia and, if uncorrected, uremia.

Testosterone and BPH

Aging and androgens are required for the development of BPH. The role of testosterone in the development of BPH has been observed since ancient times, when boys castrated before reaching puberty failed not only to attain secondary sexual characteristics but also to develop urinary obstruction in old age. Thus, castration was an early treatment for acute urinary obstruction, providing relief in about one-third of patients. For the past 50 years, the less drastic transurethral resection of the prostate has been the mainstay of treatment.

Currently, although surgery continues to be widely used, medical therapy directed at the known interaction between testosterone and prostatic growth is assuming increasing importance. Briefly, that interaction involves the following sequence (Figure 5.4):

- Luteinizing hormone (LH) stimulates the testis to secrete testosterone.
- Testosterone is converted to dihydrotestosterone (DHT) by the enzyme 5α-reductase, present in the prostate cell's cytoplasm.
- DHT binds to androgen receptor in the prostate cell.
- DHT-receptor complex enters prostate cell nucleus, where it activates DNA transcription of androgen-dependent gene.

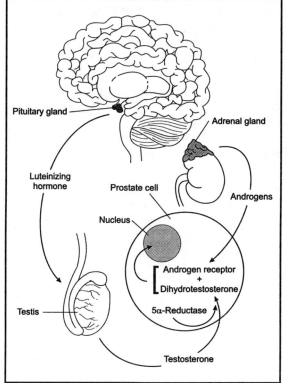

FIGURE 5.4 — TESTOSTERONE AND PROSTATIC GROWTH

Luteinizing hormone-releasing hormone stimulates the pituitary gland to release luteinizing hormone, which stimulates the testes to produce testosterone (95% of which is produced by the testes). In the prostate cell, testosterone is converted to its more active metabolite, dihydrotestosterone (DHT), by the enzyme 5α-reductase. Then DHT binds to the cytoplasmic androgen receptor and the complex enters the cell's nucleus where it activates transcription of androgen-dependent genes.

Although the role of testosterone in the development of BPH has been confirmed, serum testosterone value does not correlate with degree of hyperplasia. For example, the normal range of serum testosterone is 300 to 1100 ng/dL. However, a man with a serum level of 750 ng/dL will not necessarily have a more hyperplastic prostate than a man with a level of 350 ng/dL. Attempts to correlate BPH formation to blood or tissue levels of DHT, 5α-reductase, and cytoplasmic DHT-receptor complexes have had conflicting results.

Compounds that have been found in high levels in patients with BPH include:

- Citric acid
- Lactic acid
- Aconitic acid
- Cadmium
- Spermine
- Magnesium
- Zinc.

6 Diagnosis

Clinical evaluation of benign prostatic hyperplasia (BPH) should include:

- History
  - Frequency of urination
  - Nocturia
  - Urinary hesitancy (decreased force of stream)
  - Sense of incomplete void with post-void residual (PVR)
  - Post-void dribbling
  - Acute urinary retention
- Physical examination
- Laboratory and radiologic studies.

In addition to data regarding the patient's past medical history and current complaints, the American Urological Association Symptom Index provides valuable diagnostic information (see Chapter 7). A self-administered questionnaire containing seven questions, the Index represents the standard test with which to assess symptoms of BPH from "mild" to "severe."

Urinary Frequency

Normal bladder capacity is 300 to 500 cc, with the sensation of fullness occurring around 250 to 300 cc. In addition to incomplete emptying of the bladder caused by an obstructing prostate, frequent urination may be secondary to:

- Bladder irritability
- Urinary tract infections (UTIs)
- Bladder stones
- Neurologic disease
- Bladder neoplasm.

Urinary Hesitancy

Decreased force of urinary stream may be caused by BPH as well as by:
- Urethral stricture
- Bladder neck contracture
- Urethral valves
- Neurogenic conditions (such as diabetes mellitus).

Acute Urinary Retention

Patients with acute urinary retention are unable to pass urine and are in acute pain. The bladder is usually distended and palpable. In addition to BPH, urinary retention may be caused by:
- Prostatitis
- Urethral stricture
- Bladder neck contracture
- Medications such as:
  - α-Agonist decongestants
  - Parasympatholytics
  - Tricyclic antidepressants
  - Tranquilizers
  - Diuretics
- Alcohol.

Physical Examination

Both an abdominal and a rectal examination are required for identification of BPH. On palpation of the suprapubic area, "dull" percussion suggests a distended bladder. (Consider other causes of abdominal pain, such as cystitis, appendicitis, and diverticulitis.)

To check for PVR, have the patient void, then palpate the bladder again. For a more accurate determination of PVR, residual urine can be evacuated through a #14 or #16 catheter. Bladder ultrasonography (US) also may be performed.

Rectal Examination

The prostate is palpated with a well-lubricated, gloved index finger to examine for:
- Prostate: size, consistency, and shape
- Hyperplasia: usually a smooth, firm, elastic enlargement of the prostate
- Evidence of indurated areas, suggestive of malignancy
- Rectal sphincter tone.

■ Hyperplasia

Prostate size on rectal examination does not always correlate with degree of obstruction. Patients with enlarged prostates may be asymptomatic, whereas those without palpably gross hyperplasia may have median lobe hypertrophy or may experience dynamically induced outlet obstruction.

■ Rectal Sphincter Tone

The bulbocavernous reflex is a sharp contraction of the anal sphincter induced by squeezing of the glans penis. Rectal sphincter tone is an indirect reflection of the state of vesical innervation; a neurogenic bladder may empty incompletely.

Laboratory Examination

Laboratory examination for patients with symptoms of BPH should include:
- Urine analysis for glucose, protein, pH, occult blood, white blood cell (WBC) count
- Urine culture and sensitivity
- Sequential Multiple Analysis (SMA-6) plus creatinine to check for renal function

- Serum prostatic acid phosphatase (PAP) and prostate-specific antigen (PSA) (PSA increases 0.3 units for every gram of BPH)
- Uroflow measurement
- Urodynamics.

Uroflow

The uroflow test, usually performed in a urologist's office, requires the patient to present with a full bladder. As he voids into the uroflow meter the rate of flow is recorded. Normal values are:
- < 40 years = > 22 cc/second
- 40 to 60 years = > 18 cc/second
- > 60 years = > 13 cc/second.

Flow rates may vary slightly according to the volume of urine in the bladder.

Urodynamics

Evaluation of the neurologic and motor activity necessary for voiding is accomplished under fluoroscopic monitoring to visualize the bladder anatomy. A catheter with pressure monitors at its tip and at the bladder neck is placed via the urethra. As the bladder is filled at a constant rate with radiopaque dye, intrabladder and bladder neck pressures are monitored. Then, with the catheter still in place, the patient is asked to void. Voiding pressure is monitored while bladder, bladder neck, and prostatic fossa are visualized under fluoroscopy.

The advantages of urodynamic testing include:
- Objective documentation of bladder function
- Visualization of site and extent of bladder outlet obstruction.

Urodynamic testing's disadvantages include:
- Cost: a relatively expensive procedure that requires specialized training
- Nonphysiologic filling of bladder
- Results that often do not correlate with symptoms because of nonphysiologic variables.

Cystoscopy

With the advent of modern fiberoptic technology, cystoscopy is usually performed on an outpatient basis with local anesthesia. General anesthesia is rarely required but may be necessary for some patients, depending on age and pain threshold. As it relates to BPH, cystoscopy can:
- Provide direct visual inspection of the prostatic fossa and bladder to identify:
  - Detrusor muscle hypertrophy (trabeculation)
  - Diverticula
  - Tumors (a cause of bladder irritability)
  - Bladder stones (a cause of irritability)
- Determine the site and degree of bladder obstruction
- Indicate the length of prostatic fossa, an important technical consideration in preparation for transurethral resection of the prostate (TURP).

Radiologic Studies

Intravenous pyelography (IVP) was once the standard modality of evaluation for men with urinary outlet obstructive symptoms. It has been superseded for the most part by US of the urinary tract except in patients with hematuria associated with BPH.

■ Intravenous Pyelography

After intravenous injection of radiopaque iodine-containing contrast, the renal collecting system, ureter, and bladder can be visualized. Patients with Stage III prostatic obstruction (decompensated bladder) will have dilated, tortuous upper tracts, and a trabeculated bladder. Residual urine can be estimated on films taken after the patient voids.

Because the contrast is excreted into the renal collecting system, the test is contraindicated in patients with:

- Compromised renal function
- Dehydration
- Iodine allergies
- Multiple myeloma.

Benadryl, epinephrine, and hydrocortisone should be available to counteract unsuspected allergic reactions.

■ Ultrasonography

Ultrasonography is currently used more frequently than IVP for several reasons (Figure 6.1):

- Faster and less expensive than IVP
- No iodine necessary, obviating the risk of nephrotoxicity and allergic reaction
- Can identify masses or hydronephrosis in kidneys and upper urinary tract
- Can evaluate bladder capacity pre- and postvoid
- Rectal ultrasonography provides direct inspection of prostatic tissue as well as estimated size.

The disadvantages of US lie in its being operator-dependent and the fact that some sonograms are difficult to interpret.

> **Note**: The Public Health Service has released clinical practice guidelines for the diagnosis and treatment of BPH (Figure 6.2).

FIGURE 6.1 — IVP AND US IMAGES COMPARED

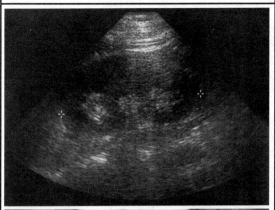

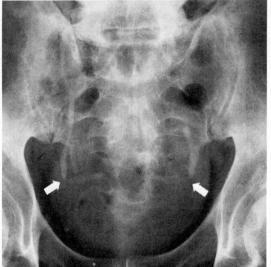

Top: Renal ultrasonogram (US) of a patient with benign prostatic hyperplasia (BPH). The kidney (between the stars) is of normal size and not hydronephrotic. *Bottom*: Intravenous pyelography (IVP) showing prominent J-hooking (shown by arrows) of ureters secondary to BPH.

FIGURE 6.2 — DIAGNOSIS/TREATMENT OF BENIGN PROSTATIC HYPERPLASIA

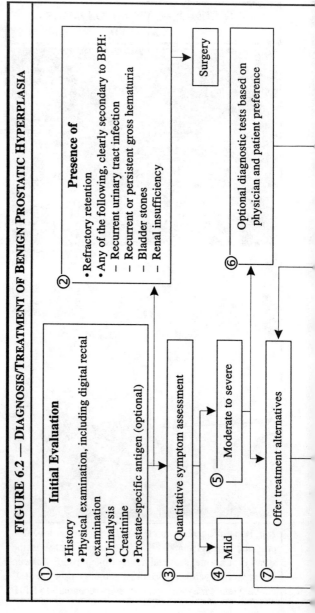

① **Initial Evaluation**
- History
- Physical examination, including digital rectal examination
- Urinalysis
- Creatinine
- Prostate-specific antigen (optional)

② **Presence of**
- Refractory retention
- Any of the following, clearly secondary to BPH:
  – Recurrent urinary tract infection
  – Recurrent or persistent gross hematuria
  – Bladder stones
  – Renal insufficiency

Surgery

③ Quantitative symptom assessment

④ Mild

⑤ Moderate to severe

⑥ Optional diagnostic tests based on physician and patient preference

⑦ Offer treatment alternatives

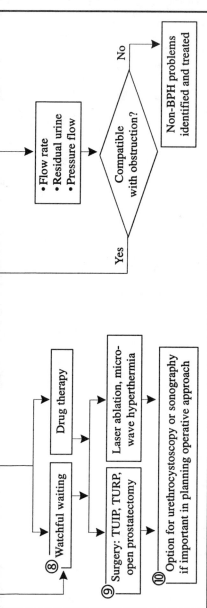

• Flow rate
• Residual urine
• Pressure flow

Compatible with obstruction?

Yes

No → Non-BPH problems identified and treated

⑧ Watchful waiting

Drug therapy

⑨ Surgery: TUIP, TURP, open prostatectomy

Laser ablation, microwave hyperthermia

⑩ Option for urethrocystoscopy or sonography if important in planning operative approach

Abbreviations: BPH, benign prostatic hyperplasia; TUIP, transurethral incision of the prostate; TURP, transurethral resection of the prostate.

This decision diagram is based on clinical practice guidelines published by the Public Health Service, US Department of Health and Human Services.

Modified and reprinted from Presti JC Jr, Stoller ML, Carroll PR. Urology. In: Tierney LM, McPhee SJ, Papadakis MA, eds. *Current Medical Diagnosis and Treatment.* Stamford, Conn: Appleton & Lange; 1996:822-857.

6

7 Treatment

Given the individual variability in benign prostatic hyperplasia's (BPH) natural history, identification of the patient who will eventually require surgery is difficult. Meanwhile, however, recent therapeutic innovations provide a range of available and future options that may defer, even prevent the need for radical surgery, including:

- Selective α-adrenergic antagonists (terazosin, doxazosin, and tamsulosin, a prostate-selective agent)
- 5α-reductase antagonists (finasteride)
- Prostatic stenting
- Microwave hyperthermia
- Visual laser ablation of the prostate
- High-intensity focused ultrasound
- Transurethral incision of the prostate (TUIP).

Indications for surgery include:
- Acute urinary retention
- Bilateral hydronephrosis (suggests Stage III obstruction)
- Chronic urinary tract infection (UTI) exacerbated by residual urine (must rule out renal stones, prostatitis)
- Bladder diverticula/stones.

Once the absolute indications for surgery are ruled out, the patient should be counseled regarding the therapeutic options. The physician may wish to suggest minor lifestyle changes, such as a decreased liquid intake and no diuretics after dinner, with a follow-up appointment scheduled in 6 to 8 weeks.

After reassurance that BPH is a common problem and a few lifestyle changes, many patients find their symptoms to be manageable without therapeutic intervention. Others find the urinary frequency and nocturia annoying and disruptive. These are the men for whom current, pharmacologic or noninvasive therapy is designed.

The American Urological Association Symptom Index may be useful in determining the most appropriate course of therapy for patients with symptoms of varying degrees but who do not require surgery (Table 7.1) Patients with scores of 0 to 7 are good candidates for watchful waiting with periodic reevaluations. Most of those with moderate (8 to 19) or severe (20 to 25) will probably be open to some form of noninvasive therapeutic intervention.

Drug Therapy

■ Alpha-adrenergic Blocking Agents

The dynamic component of BPH reflects the tone or degree of contraction of prostate smooth muscle, which is found in hyperplastic tissue as well as the capsule. A rich supply of α-adrenergic receptors has been demonstrated in the prostate, along with few β-adrenergic and barely detectable cholinergic receptors. The bladder neck, unlike the bladder itself, is also well endowed with α-adrenergic receptors.

Two types of α-adrenergic receptors are present in the prostate, α_1 and α_2. Three subtypes of the α_1 receptor have been identified in prostatic tissue, with α_{1A} responsible for contraction of prostatic smooth muscle. Thus, selective α_1-adrenergic-antagonist agents should decrease bladder resistance to urinary outflow. And because of the relative sparsity of α-adrenergic receptors in the bladder proper, its contraction should be unaffected. Selective α_1-adrenergic blockade has become the medical treatment of first choice for BPH (Table 7.2).

The currently approved drugs include (Figure 7.1):
- Terazosin (Hytrin)
- Doxazosin (Cardura)
- Tamsulosin (Flomax), a new prostate-selective α_{1A}-adrenoceptor antagonist.

Terazosin Hydrochloride (Hytrin)

Initially used as an antihypertensive, terazosin is currently indicated for BPH as well. This selective α_1-adrenergic blocker is characterized by:
- A half-life of approximately 12 hours (14 hours for men > 70 years of age and 11 hours for those 20 to 39 years old), allowing once-a-day dosing
- Approximately 40% of administered dose is excreted in the urine, 60% in the feces; impaired renal function has no significant effect on elimination
- Small but significant decreases in total cholesterol and combined low-density lipoprotein (LDL)/very low-density lipoprotein (VLDL) fractions, with no significant changes in high-density lipoprotein (HDL) and triglycerides.

According to clinical trials of terazosin in men with symptomatic BPH:
- Approximately 70% of patients experience improvement in symptoms
- Mean improvement in obstructive and irritative symptoms of 62% and 31%, respectively
- Peak and mean urinary flow rates improved 31% and 47%, respectively
- Symptom scores and peak urine flow rates significantly improved from baseline by week 2.

TABLE 7.1 — AMERICAN UROLOGICAL ASSOCIATION SYMPTOM INDEX FOR BENIGN PROSTATIC HYPERPLASIA

Questions to be Answered	Not at all	Less than One Time in Five	Less Than Half the Time	About Half the Time	More Than Half the Time	Almost Always
1. Over the past month, how often have you had a sensation of not emptying your bladder completely after you finish urinating?	0	1	2	3	4	5
2. Over the past month, how often have you had to urinate again less than 2 hours after you finished urinating?	0	1	2	3	4	5
3. Over the past month, how often have you found you stopped and started again several times when you urinated?	0	1	2	3	4	5
4. Over the past month, how often have you found it difficult to postpone urination?	0	1	2	3	4	5

	0	1	2	3	4	5
5. Over the past month, how often have you had a weak urinary stream?	0	1	2	3	4	5
6. Over the past month, how often have you had to push or strain to begin urination?	0	1	2	3	4	5
7. Over the past month, how many times did you most typically get up to urinate from the time you went to bed at night until the time you got up in the morning?	0	1	2	3	4	5

Sum of seven circled numbers equals the symptom score. See text for explanation.

Reproduced with permission from Barry MJ, Fowler FJ Jr, O'Leary MP, et al. The American Urological Association symptom index for benign prostatic hyperplasia. The Measurement Committee of the American Urological Association. *J Urol*. 1992;148:1549-1557.

7

TABLE 7.2 — DRUG THERAPY FOR BENIGN PROSTATIC HYPERPLASIA

Agent	Dose	Action	Laboratory Results	Side Effects
Terazosin	Initial: 1 mg, hs; titrate to 2, 5, or 10 mg, qd	α_1-Adrenoceptor blocker; relaxes prostate smooth muscle; decreases mean diastolic blood pressure: 15.1 mm Hg – hypertensives 2.2 mm Hg – normotensives 1.8 mm Hg – controlled hypertension	No effect on prostate-specific antigen (PSA)	Dizziness, asthenia, somnolence, postural hypotension if taken with other htn medication, esp. calcium-channel blocker
Doxazosin	Initial: 1 mg, AM or PM; titrate over 1 to 2 weeks to 2 mg, 4 mg, 8 mg	α_1-Adrenoceptor blocker relaxes prostate smooth muscle; decreases mean diastolic blood pressure: 8.0 mm Hg – hypertensives 2.6 mm Hg – normotensives	No effect on PSA	Fatigue, dizziness
Tamulosin	0.4 mg, once/day	α_{1A}-Adrenoceptor blocker; prostate selective; no clinically relevant blood pressure reduction	No effect on PSA	Abnormal ejaculation
Finasteride	5 mg, once/day	5α-Reductase inhibitor; reduces prostate volume	PSA decreases (with prostate volume)	Impotence, decreased libido; decreased volume of ejaculate

FIGURE 7.1 — THE α_1-SELECTIVE ADRENOCEPTOR BLOCKERS

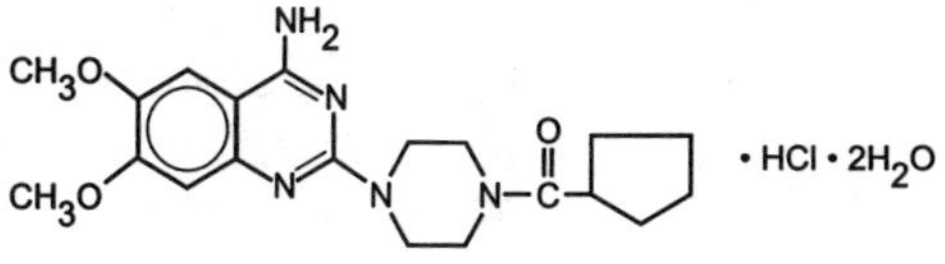

Terazosin (Hytrin)

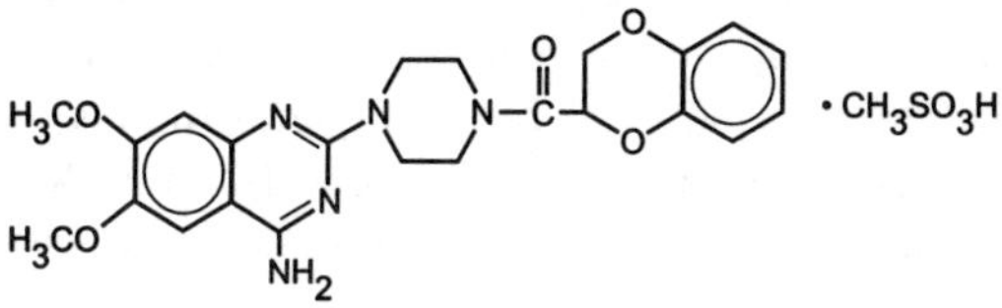

Doxazosin (Cardura)

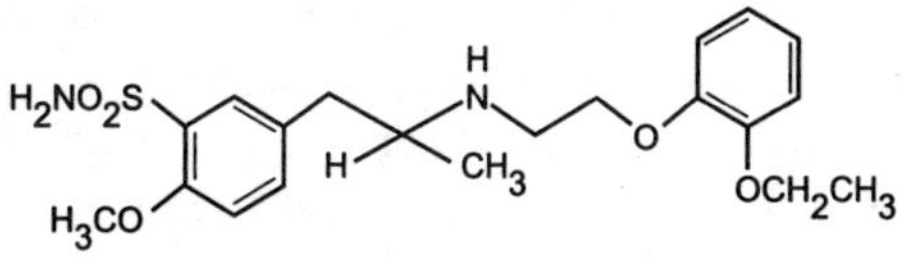

Tamsulosin (Flomax)

Shown here are the comparative structures of terazosin, doxazosin, and tamsulosin.

Side Effects

According to the results of six placebo-controlled trials of terazosin in BPH, the adverse reactions that were significantly more common in patients receiving terazosin than in those receiving placebo included:

- Asthenia: terazosin, 7.4% vs placebo, 3.3%
- Postural hypotension: 3.9% vs 0.8%
- Dizziness: 9.1% vs 4.2%
- Somnolence: 3.6% vs 1.9%

- Nasal congestion (rhinitis): 1.9% vs 0.0%
- Impotence: 1.6% vs 0.6%.

Although terazosin lowers blood pressure in hypertensive patients with increased peripheral resistance, normotensive men do not experience a clinically significant blood pressure-lowering effect.

Analysis of the incidence rate of hypotensive adverse events adjusted for length of treatment has shown the risk to be greatest during the initial 7 days of treatment, although it continues throughout the therapeutic course. When using terazosin and other antihypertensive agents concomitantly, dosage reduction and retitration of either agent may be necessary.

Dosage

The initial dose of terazosin is 1 mg at bedtime to minimize the risk of a severe hypotensive response, followed by titration up to 2, 5, or 10 mg once a day.

Doses of 5 mg to 10 mg are usually required for clinical response, with a 4- to 6-week course required to assess achievement of a beneficial response.

Doxazosin Mesylate (Cardura)

The only other selective α_1-adrenoceptor antagonist currently indicated for BPH as well as hypertension, doxazosin is structurally and pharmacologically similar to terazosin. (Its half-life is longer, however, at 22 hours.) For example:

- Similar pharmacokinetics in men < 65 years of age and those ≥ 65 for plasma half-life values and oral clearance
- No significant pharmacokinetic alterations in elderly patients and patients with renal impairment compared to younger patients with normal renal function

- Small reductions in total serum cholesterol (2% to 3%) and LDL cholesterol (4%) and a small increase in HDL/total cholesterol ratio (4%) in normocholesterolemic patients.

Results of a number of clinical trials of doxazosin in the treatment of BPH have demonstrated:
- Improvements in symptoms and maximum urinary flow rate experienced by 66% to 71% of patients
- Significant relief seen as early as 1 week into treatment regimen
- Both hypertension and BPH can be treated with doxazosin monotherapy.

Side Effects

Adverse reactions experienced among at least 1% of 965 men being treated for BPH alone (doxazosin, 5 mg to 8 mg) or for BPH plus hypertension (1 mg to 16 mg), which reached significance compared with placebo, were:
- Fatigue: 8.0% vs 1.7%
- Hypotension: 1.7% vs 0.0%
- Edema: 2.7% vs 0.7%
- Dizziness: 15.6% vs 9.0%
- Dyspnea: 2.6% vs 0.3%.

Dizziness and dyspnea appeared to be dose-related.

Treatment of normotensive men with BPH did not result in a clinically significant blood pressure-lowering effect.

Dosage

The initial dose is 1 mg, once daily in morning or evening, to minimize the frequency of postural hypotension and first-dose syncope associated with the doxazosin.

During a titration interval of 1 to 2 weeks, including routine blood pressure evaluations, dosage may be increased to 2 mg, then 4 mg. The usually recommended dose for BPH is 2 mg to 4 mg, depending on efficacy.

Tamsulosin Hydrochloride (Flomax)

This most recently approved α_1-adrenoceptor antagonist, unlike terazosin and doxazosin, is highly selective for the α_1-adrenoceptor subtype, α_{1A}, which is predominant and functional in the human prostate. In fact, tamsulosin is about 12 times more selective for the α_1-adrenoceptors in the human prostate than those in the aorta.

According to meta-analysis of two European randomized, multicenter studies in patients with symptomatic BPH, tamsulosin is as effective as both terazosin and doxazosin in the treatment of symptomatic BPH but has only a minor effect on blood pressure and causes fewer vasodilatory side effects.

According to two 13-week US studies, patients treated with the standard therapeutic dose of tamsulosin, 0.4 mg/day, showed a 5.1 to 8.3 point reduction from pretreatment baseline in the American Urological Association's (AUA) 35-point scale, beginning only 1 week after starting treatment. Symptom scores remained decreased through 13 weeks in both studies. The group of study patients who received 0.8 mg/day (recommended for men who show no response to the standard dose after 2 to 4 weeks) experienced a slightly greater decline in AUA score, between 5.8 and 9.6. Tamsulosin's advantages include:

- Rapid decrease in symptoms starting 1 week after dosing
- Significant increase in urine flow 4 to 8 hours after the first dose

- Treatment can be initiated with the full therapeutic dose, with minimal risk of symptomatic postural hypotension and syncope
- Gradual titration of dosage unnecessary.

Adverse Reactions

In the European studies, side effects commonly associated with non-subtype-selective α_1-adrenoceptor antagonists (dizziness, postural hypotension, syncope, and asthenia) were low in tamsulosin patients and not different from the placebo group. The only adverse event that occurred in significantly more tamsulosin than placebo patients was abnormal ejaculation (4.5% and 1%, respectively).

In the US studies, abnormal ejaculation was reported in 8.4% of the 0.4 mg/day group, 18.1% in the 0.8 mg group, and 0.2% in controls. However, there were no patient withdrawals in the 0.4 mg or placebo groups and only 8 (1.6%) of 492 patients in the 0.8 mg group.

Abnormal ejaculation has been reported with other α_1-adrenoceptor antagonists at a similar rate of 4% to 11%. Generally noticed as retrograde ejaculation or a decreased volume of ejaculate, the phenomenon may be related to the agents' mode of action: relaxation of smooth muscle in the bladder neck and prostatic urethra, as well as in the vas deferens and seminal vesicles.

■ Androgen-deprivation Agents

Finasteride (Proscar), a synthetic inhibitor of the testosterone-converting enzyme 5α-reductase, blocks the effect of dihydrotestosterone (DHT) on the prostate's DNA effectively reducing the size of the prostate. It has minimal effects on libido or sexual function, improves maximum flow rates, and slows the progression of BPH.

The first 5α-reductase inhibitor to undergo clinical testing, finasteride is also the only such agent of its kind (Table 7.2). Its pharmacologic and physiologic characteristics include:

- A 90% decrease in prostatic DHT levels (by doses of 1 mg to 100 mg)
- A mean serum half-life of 8 hours in elderly men (6 hours in middle-aged patients) and an even longer biologic half-life, allowing once-a-day dosage of 5 mg
- No dosage adjustment required in patients with renal impairment (decrease in urinary excretion associated with increased fecal excretion)
- Although prostatic testosterone is increased about seven-fold, serum testosterone rises but only within normal limits
- No effect on serum lipids or bone density.

According to clinical trials of finasteride in men with symptomatic BPH:

- An estimated 30% to 50% of patients will respond to treatment
- Prostate volume is reduced by approximately 20%
- Maximum urinary flow rate and symptom scores are improved
- Finasteride can reverse the natural progression of BPH
- Improvement is sometimes seen by 1 month, but finasteride must be taken for 6 to 12 months to obtain maximum effect.

A recent study designed to identify pretreatment predictors of outcome (expressed by symptoms or peak urinary flow rates) concluded that the difference in magnitude of improvement between finasteride and placebo *becomes significant for men with a prostate volume greater than 40 cc. Thus, men with smaller organs may not be suitable candidates for finasteride therapy.*

Side Effects
Finasteride's only important side effects are:
- Impotence (reported by 3.7%)
- Decreased libido (3.3%)
- Decreased volume of ejaculate (2.8%).

This suggests that a small percentage of men may require DHT as well as testosterone for normal sexual function.

Prostate-specific Antigen Screening
Prostate-specific antigen (PSA) is a glycoprotein produced only by prostate epithelial cells, which hydrolyzes the coagulum of the ejaculate. Since serum PSA concentration correlates with prostate size (and size with age), levels generally decrease in patients treated with finasteride. Within the first months of therapy, PSA levels usually stabilize to about half of pretreatment values. Thus, by 6 months, screening values should be doubled for comparison to normal ranges in untreated men. Because of the effect of finasteride on PSA, it may be more difficult to detect prostate cancer in these patients.

The effect of long-term finasteride therapy on occult prostate carcinoma is unknown. However, the National Cancer Institute's Prostate Cancer Prevention Trial is currently underway to determine if inhibition of DHT synthesis in the prostate over a prolonged period will lead to a decreased incidence of prostate cancer. The multicenter study involves 18,000 men older than 55 years of age who will be randomized to receive finasteride or placebo. Cell proliferation experiments *in vitro* have shown the growth rate of a human carcinoma cell line to be dose-dependently inhibited by both finasteride and antiandrogens.

■ **Transurethral Incision of the Prostate**

Transurethral incision of the prostate may be performed in patients with bladder-outlet obstruction and small prostates weighing 30 g or less.

Following cystoscopic examination to evaluate prostate size, degree of obstruction and incidental pathology, the urologist uses a cutting electrode to:

- Make incisions at the 5- and 7-o'clock positions, extending across bladder neck and prostatic urethra to the verumontanum
- Incisions are deepened until capsular fibers are in view
- Prostatic lobes fall away as capsule is incised, probably due to incision of muscle fibers (Figure 7.2).

Possible complications of TUIP include:
- Retrograde ejaculation
- Scarring may lead to recurrence of symptoms.

■ **Transurethral Resection of the Prostate**

Indications for transurethral resection of the prostate (TURP) include:

- Progressive symptoms with significant outlet obstruction
- Significant post-void residual (PVR)
- Urinary retention (with failed voiding trials)
- Recurrent UTIs due to retained urine
- Bladder stones
- Recurrent hematuria due to prostatic bleeding
- Azotemia/uremia secondary to obstruction.

The prostate itself can be compared to an orange, with its pulp the hyperplastic tissue and its peel the capsule. Transurethral prostatectomy resects only the

FIGURE 7.2 — TRANSURETHRAL INCISION OF THE PROSTATE

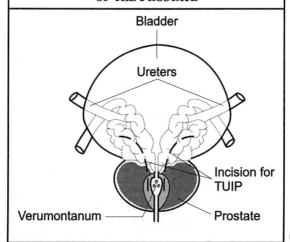

Transurethral incision of the prostate (TUIP) usually involves two incisions made with a cutting electrode at the 5- and 7-o'clock positions, begun distal to the interureteric ridge and extended across the bladder neck and prostatic urethra to the verumontanum. As the incisions are deepened, the bladder neck and prostatic urethra spring open to relieve the bladder-outlet obstruction.

pulp, leaving the capsule as the conduit between bladder and urethra. The endoscopic procedure:

- Is performed in the operating room under spinal or general anesthesia
- The resectoscope is initially placed into the bladder and the bladder is inspected for abnormalities
- Care is taken to identify the ureteral orifices and their position relative to the bladder neck
- Tissue is resected with a cautery loop passed through the resectoscope into the bladder (Figure 7.3)

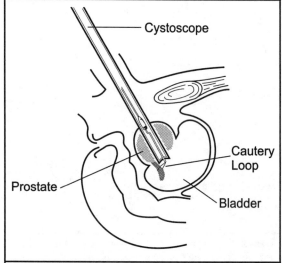

FIGURE 7.3 — TRANSURETHRAL RESECTION OF THE PROSTATE

In this lateral view of transurethral resection of the prostate (TURP), the cystoscope is placed into the bladder and "chips" of the hyperplastic prostate are resected with a cautery loop.

- Throughout surgery, prostatic "chips" are irrigated out of bladder and sent to pathology
- Surgery generally limited to 1 hour to prevent overabsorption of irrigant with resultant hyponatremia
- After the procedure, a Foley catheter is left in place for 2 or 3 days.

TURP has been associated with both early and late complications.
- Early:
  - Hyponatremia
  - Failure to void
  - Persistent bleeding/clot retention

- Late:
  - Recurrent BPH
  - Bladder neck contracture
  - Urethral stricture
  - Mild stress incontinence
  - Impotence.

In summary, TURP has been shown to be an effective treatment for urinary retention with low morbidity and mortality (0.2%). It is, however, a surgical procedure with associated risks and expense. Patients should be carefully evaluated and informed of alternative treatment options. Open (supra- or retropubic) prostatectomy is performed only in patients with extremely large prostate glands that would require prolonged surgery.

■ Transurethral Vaporization of the Prostate

A new technique, transurethral vaporization of the prostate (TUVP) involves a grooved roller electrode, pure-cutting diathermy, and a standard irrigating resectoscope to rapidly heat prostatic tissue to $> 100°$ C, resulting in vaporization and cavitation of the prostatic adenoma. The procedure takes 20 to 65 minutes, and most patients have their catheters removed within 24 hours and are discharged on the second day after treatment. Symptom scores improve by 67% and residual volumes by 72%.

Minimally Invasive Treatments

■ Prostatic Stents

Stenting is usually reserved for patients with multiple medical problems that prohibit additional medication or surgical intervention for BPH. Two types of stent are currently available: a flexible, self-expanding (to 1.4 cm) prosthesis made of a nonmagnetic superalloy woven into a tubular mesh; and an inert titanium device that can be expanded to 1.1 cm (but is not self-expanding). A new thermoexpansible permanent stent is under clinical investigation in Europe.

The advantages of prostatic stents include:

- Quick placement (15 minutes or less) under regional anesthesia
- Minimal intraoperative and postoperative bleeding
- Patient can be discharged same day or next morning
- Do not alter serum concentration of PSA.

Disadvantages include:
- Prepositioning may be difficult
- Sometimes cause irritation and urinary frequency
- May migrate, causing pain and/or incontinence
- Removal can be difficult, may be required in > one-third of patients.

According to one study of long-term (63 months) prostatic stent placement for BPH, the prostheses can be effective in relieving bladder outlet obstruction caused by BPH. However, they appear to be most useful in patients at high surgical risk and with a limited life expectancy. The investigators recommend the procedure primarily for patients who would otherwise be treated with an indwelling catheter.

■ **Laser Therapy**
Laser coagulation prostatectomy with the neodymium:yttrium-argon-garnet (Nd:YAG) wavelength, or visual laser ablation of the prostate (VLAP), has now been studied in patients with BPH long enough to be considered an efficacious surgical intervention with minimal associated morbidity. Voiding outcomes have been found to persist through 3 years.

Excess or resectable BPH tissue is estimated based on combined cystoscopic appearance and digital palpation before treatment. The laser fiber is positioned in the prostatic urethra under direct vision through the working channel of a standard 21 to 22 French cystoscope. The procedure involves fixed spot laser applications, spatially separated by no more than 1 to 2 cm along lateral and median lobes, to produce coagulation necrosis in all obstructing tissue (Figure 7.4).

Some comparative outcome results in laser and transurethral prostatectomy include:

- Improvements in symptom scores, peak urinary flow, and PVR similar for both procedures
- No significant incidence of bleeding complications and, in turn, a zero incidence of transfusion in VLAP patients compared to 5% to 10% associated with TURP
- No stress urinary incontinence in laser-treated patients compared to 2% in TURP
- Late occurring urethral stricture 1.8% in VLAP compared to 16% in TURP (difference probably due to VLAP's shorter operative times and smaller caliber cystoscopes and catheters)
- Incidence of bladder neck strictures similar in two procedures, may be reduced in VLAP if high-power treatments avoided
- 5.3% incidence of reoperation for residual tissue at median follow-up > 2 years similar for both procedures
- VLAP has improved voiding outcomes in men with prostates $\geq$ 80 gm in size (although significantly less than in those with smaller prostates), most of which would be considered unsuitable for TURP.

FIGURE 7.4 — LASER COAGULATION OF PROSTATIC HYPERPLASIA

Urolase Laser Prostatectomy – Lateral Lobes

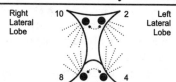

Four Quadrant Spot Applications

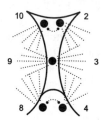

"Sextant" Approach to Larger Glands

Urolase Laser Prostatectomy – Median Lobe

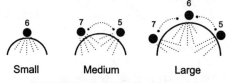

| Small | Medium | Large |

Each Application: 40 watts × 90 seconds

The operative approach to laser coagulation of BPH involves continuous 90-second fixed spot applications of Nd:YAG laser energy to the lateral and median lobes of hyperplasia. Depending on prostate size, 40 watt spot applications are made at four (2, 4, 8 and 10 o'clock) or six (2, 3, 4, 8, 9 and 10 o'clock) positions to the lateral lobes and at 6 o'clock; 5 and 7 o'clock; or 5, 6 and 7 o'clock to the median lobe.

Adapted from Kabalin JN, Bite G, Doll S. Neodymium:YAG laser coagulation prostatectomy: 3 years experience with 227 patients. *J Urol*. 1996;155:182.

■ Transurethral Microwave Thermotherapy (Prostatron)

In this procedure, temperatures of 41 to 44° C are delivered to the prostate by either a transrectal or urethral probe. The effects of hyperthermia on BPH include:

- Minimal decrease of prostatic volume
- Minimal tissue necrosis
- No change in PSA value.

Suggested mechanisms of action are:

- Loss of androgen receptors
- Change in α-adrenergic tone of capsular smooth muscle.

According to a 1995 multicenter study of changes in pressure-flow parameters by transurethral microwave thermotherapy in men with BPH, the procedure appears to affect bladder outlet obstruction differently than TURP. In thermotherapy, a minor change in voiding detrusor pressures occurs in the absence of significant tissue loss and cavity formation. The increased urinary flow rates observed after microwave heating depend on greater elasticity of the prostatic urethra. Thus, hyperthermia seems to be selectively successful in patients with predominantly constrictive obstruction (Figure 7.5). Such patients can be identified only by pressure-flow studies, however.

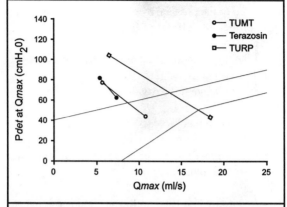

FIGURE 7.5 — COMPARATIVE EFFICACY OF TUMT, TURP AND TERAZOSIN

Comparison of the effects of high energy transurethral microwave thermotherapy (TUMT), transurethral prostatectomy (TURP), and terazosin therapy on moderate to severe bladder outlet obstruction shows the improvement after TUMT to be in the range of (although not equal to) that after TURP and significantly greater than noted after medication.

Abbreviations: P*det* at Q*max* (cmH$_2$O), mean detrusor pressure; Q*max*, maximum flow.

Adapted from de la Rosette JJ, de Wildt MJ, Höfner K, Carter SS, Debruyne FM, Tubaro A. Pressure-flow study analyses in patients treated with high energy thermotherapy. *J Urol*. 1996; 156:1428-1433.

PART 4

PROSTATE CANCER

8 Prostate Cancer

Cancer of the prostate is the most common cancer in American males. Optimal management of patients with prostate and other urologic malignancies requires close cooperation between the primary-care physician, urologist, surgeon, radiologist, and medical oncologist. Contributions from each member of this team have produced advances in diagnosis, staging, and therapy, all of which have improved survival and quality of life for many of these patients.

Epidemiology

- Cancer of the prostate was diagnosed in more than 300,000 men in 1996 and was the second leading cause of death among men who die of cancer.
- Prostate cancer represents 20% of all newly diagnosed malignancies.
- In 1995, prostate cancer accounted for 12.3% of cancer deaths in men.
- Prostate cancer is the most common malignant disorder in African-American men and the second most common cause of death from cancer in this group.
- The probability of developing prostate cancer is higher among African-American men (9.4%) than in Caucasian men (8.7%).
- Incidence of clinical prostate cancer is 30% in men 70 to 79 years of age, 67% in those 80 to 89 years old.
- 30% to 50% of patients have invasive or metastatic disease on initial presentation.

- The incidence of clinical prostate cancer is much lower in Asian men, suggesting environmental and/or dietary factors may influence its development.

Etiology

Despite the high incidence of prostate cancer, little is understood about how and why it develops except that its occurrence depends on the presence of testosterone. Males castrated before puberty are not at risk for either cancer or benign hyperplasia of the prostate.

Possible etiologies include:
- A diet high in saturated fatty acids
- Genetic factors (familial, racial predilection; suppressor gene mutation)
- Exposure to environmental toxins, heavy metals (ie, cadmium)
- Viral infection (may act as initiator).

A relationship between benign prostatic hyperplasia (BPH) and prostate cancer is controversial. Although both depend on testosterone, mechanisms of initiation and progression are not directly related to testosterone concentration. The processes are probably unrelated. However, the presence of BPH may make the clinical diagnosis of prostate cancer more difficult.

Natural History

Prostate cancer is primarily a disease of older men, uncommon in men under age 50. The course of the disease is variable. It usually starts as a single focus in the peripheral zone of the prostate, although a small percentage of malignancies arise in the central (5% to 10%) and transition zones (20%) (Figure 8.1).

FIGURE 8.1 — DIAGRAM OF PROSTATE AND URETHRA IN SIDE VIEW

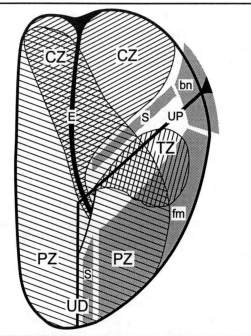

This diagram of prostate and urethra in side view locates the proximal (UP) and distal (UD) segments of the prostatic urethra and the ejaculatory ducts (E) in relation to the anteromedial nonglandular tissues: bladder neck (bn); anterior fibromuscular stroma (fm); preprostatic sphincter (s); distal striated sphincter (s). These structures, in turn, are shown in relation to a three-dimensional representation of the zones of the glandular prostate: central zone (CZ); peripheral zone (PZ); transitional zone (TZ). The majority of prostate cancers arise in the peripheral zone, 20% in the transitional zone, and 5% to 10% in the central zone.

From Stamey TA, McNeal JE. Adenocarcinoma of the prostate. In: Walsh PC, Retik AB, Stamey TA, eds. *Cambell's Urology*. Volume 2. Philadelphia, Pa: WB Saunders Co; 1992:1159-1221.

In prostate cancer, unlike other cancers, it is often assumed that most localized disease will have little or no effect on the quality or duration of life. This difference in perspective has arisen because of the uniquely high prevalence of undiagnosed prostate cancer in men older than 50 years. Autopsy prevalence of prostatic carcinoma reaches:

- 30% in the seventh decade
- 40% in the eighth decade
- 50% in the ninth decade.

An estimated 1.05% of the total population reservoir of cancer reaches clinical diagnosis in any year, and given the total prevalence of histologic cancer, the annual mortality rate is only 0.31%.

The prolonged natural history of prostate cancer in the absence of interventional therapy, especially in the early clinical stages, is evident in the following examples of data regarding progression:

- More than two-thirds of all clinical stage A and B cancers (organ confined, see *Diagnosis*) take in excess of 4 years to double
- In patients younger than 70 years of age with clinical stage B disease, cumulative 5- and 10-year probability for:
  - Progression to stage C (locally invasive) was 49% and 79%, respectively
  - Developing metastases, 8% and 23%, respectively
  - Dying of prostate cancer, 2% and 8%, respectively
- Ten-year follow-up of 29 men with palpable clinical stage B tumors (20 of whom were "expectantly" treated) found:
  - Three had died of prostatic cancer
  - Six had developed metastases.

9 Diagnosis

Prostate cancer does not usually cause symptoms until it has become locally invasive or metastatic. Symptoms may include:
- Urinary frequency and obstruction because of local tumor mass
- Pelvic lymph node metastases that may cause leg edema
- Bone pain (bone metastases).

The digital rectal examination (DRE) and serum prostate-specific antigen (PSA) level are the primary diagnostic tools. Benign tissue is soft, like the thenar eminence of the thumb, whereas cancer is:
- Firm
- Indurated
- Asymmetrical
- Stony (like the bridge of the nose).

Most peripheral or central zone cancers and those in the transition zone benign prostatic hyperplasia (BPH) area are not palpable by DRE. Other factors that may distort rectal examination include:
- Very large prostate (BPH)
- Prostatitis
- Prostatic calculi
- Focal infarction
- Prior biopsies or transurethral prostatectomy.

Serum Markers

A major factor in the increased detection of prostate cancer is the widespread use of serum PSA screening. PSA is a glycoprotein produced only by prostate epithelial cells, which hydrolyzes the coagulum of the ejaculate. Unique among tumor markers, PSA rises at an overall average rate of 3.5 ng/mL per gram of intracapsular cancer regardless of extracapsular penetration. (In BPH, PSA levels are elevated by only 0.3 ng/mL per gram, and the rise in levels over time is much less steep than in cancer: 3.0 to 3.4 ng/mL in BPH vs 4.2 to 14 ng/mL in cancer.)

Before the introduction of PSA, serum prostatic acid phosphatase (PAP) and radioimmunoassay for human PAP (RIA-PAP) were the standard markers for prostate cancer. However, PAP is significantly elevated only in patients with metastatic disease. Therefore it is not a good predictor of early malignancies within the gland itself. Furthermore, BPH causes elevations of RIA-PAP in 14% of patients, primarily in those with greater than 40 g of benign hyperplasia.

Tissue Biopsy

Once a suspicious DRE is noted or an elevated PSA value obtained, the prostate should be biopsied, using a transrectal ultrasound (TRUS) guided procedure. Aspirin, alcohol, or nonsteroidal anti-inflammatory medications should not be taken by the patient for 1 week prior to the biopsy.

■ TRUS-guided Biopsy

Patients are required to have a Fleets enema and to take an oral antibiotic (ciprofloxacin, 500 mg bid, or equivalent) for 1 day before and 2 days after the procedure.

With the patient lying on his side, the rectal probe is inserted, the nodule is localized on both transverse and longitudinal planes, and the biopsy is performed with a needle inserted through a port in the probe.

The advantages of this procedure are:
- It is less painful
- It achieves direct sampling of prostatic tissue
- It can examine periprostatic, seminal vesicle, or bladder invasion by the tumor, and any suspicious areas can be biopsied as well.

The disadvantages are:
- Possible infection with rectal bacteria
- Excessive bleeding may be difficult to control.

The possible complications of TRUS-guided biopsy include:
- Rectal injury
- Sepsis
- Urethral injury
- Hematuria
- Urinary retention.

Histology

Histologic grading of prostate cancer can be difficult because distinct architectural patterns are often found in different areas of the same tumor. The grading system most commonly used by pathologists, the Gleason Sum System, handles this problem by assigning a "primary" grade to the cancer pattern occupying the greatest area of the specimen and a "secondary" grade to that in the second largest area.

The Gleason Sum System is based on five patterns of prostate cancer that represent a continuum of dedifferentiation (Figure 9.1). As the newly formed malignant cells lose their ability to form normal glands, the cancer's grade of severity increases. Gleason scores can be divided into:
- Well differentiated: Gleason 2, 3, 4 (1+1, 1+2, 2+2)

① Sharply circumscribed aggregate of small, closely packed, uniform glands

② Greater variation in glandular size

More stroma between glands

More infiltrative margins

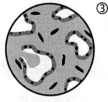

③ Further variation in glandular size

Glands more widely dispersed in stroma

Distinctly infiltrative margins, with loss of circumscription

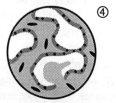

④ "Fused gland" pattern; irregular masses of neoplastic glands coalescing and branching

Infiltration of prostatic stroma

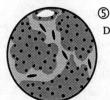

⑤ Diffusely infiltrating tumor cells with only occasional gland formation

Prominent nucleoli

The two predominant patterns of tumor architecture at low-power magnification are added for a "sum" score, eg: ② + ③ = 5.

- Moderately differentiated: Gleason 5, 6, 7
- Poorly differentiated: Gleason 8, 9, 10.

The poorly differentiated cancers are more likely to spread to the prostate and involve lymph nodes. Lymphatic spread includes:
- Obturator nodes
- Internal iliac nodes
- Common iliac nodes
- Presacral nodes
- Para-aortic nodes.

Hematogenous metastases occur to bone more frequently than to viscera, and diffuse pulmonary involvement is infrequent.

Staging

Once the diagnosis of prostate cancer is made by biopsy, the extent of tumor spread must be evaluated. Two staging systems are currently available: the TNM (tumor, nodes and metastases) classification of the American Joint Cancer Committee (Table 9.1) which is the most widely used system; and the system devised by the Organ Systems Coordinating Center of the National Cancer Institute and published by W.F. Whitmore, Jr. (Table 9.2). Prostate cancer is defined by the following four stages:
- T1: nonpalpable, detected by PSA or DRE
- T2: detected by DRE
- T3: extends outside the prostate capsule
- T4: invades surrounding organs.

Figure 9.2 illustrates the palpable findings on DRE for Whitmore clinical stages TA, TB, and TC.

TABLE 9.1 — TNM STAGING SYSTEM FOR PROSTATE CANCER

T: *Primary Tumor*	
Tx	Cannot be assessed
T0	No evidence of primary tumor
Tis	Carcinoma *in situ* (CIS)
T1a	$\leq$ 3 foci of carcinoma in resection for benign disease; normal digital rectal examination
T1b	$\geq$ 3 foci of carcinoma in resection for benign disease; normal digital rectal examination
T1c	Detected from elevated PSA alone; normal digital rectal examination
T2a	Tumor in less than half of one lobe
T2b	Tumor in more than half of one lobe
T2c	Tumor in both lobes
T3a	Unilateral extracapsular extension
T3b	Bilateral extracapsular extension
T3c	Seminal vesicle involvement
T4	Adjacent organ involvement
N: *Regional Lymph Nodes*	
Nx	Cannot be assessed
N0	No regional lymph node metastasis
N1	Metastasis in single lymph node $\leq$ 2 cm
N2	Metastasis in a single lymph node > 2 cm and < 5 cm or multiple nodes none > 5 cm
N3	Metastasis in lymph node > 5 cm
M: *Distant Metastasis*	
Mx	Cannot be assessed
M0	No distant metastasis
M1	Distant metastasis present

Abbreviations: TNM; tumor, nodes and metastases.

TABLE 9.2 — ORGAN SYSTEMS COORDINATING CENTER CLASSIFICATION FOR CLINICAL STAGING OF PROSTATE CANCER

T: *Primary Tumor*

TX	Anatomic relationships indefinable (eg, prior total prostatectomy)
TA	Digitally unrecognizable cancer (confirmed histologically and substaged if traditional TUR cancer)
TA1	≤ 5% of total surgical specimen and of low to medium grade
TA2	> 5% of specimen, any grade, or ≤ 5% of specimen with any high grade
TAX	TA, but not A1 or A2
TB	Digitally palpated cancer, organ-confined
TB1	≤ ½ of one lobe, regardless of location
TB2	> ½ of one lobe but not > 1 lobe
TB3	> 1 lobe or bilaterally palpable cancer
TBX	Palpable, organ-confined cancer, not otherwise characterized
TBC*	Palpable cancer extending beyond prostate capsule
TC1	Extension beyond margin unilaterally (may include seminal vesicle)
TC2	Extension bilaterally (may include seminal vesicle)
TC3	Extension into bladder, rectum, levator muscles, or pelvic side walls

N: *Lymph Node Status*

N0 (C/H)	No regional lymph node metastases, clinically (C) and/or histologically (H)

Continued

N1 (C/H)	Microscopic regional lymph node metastasis, proved histologically
N2 (C/H)	Gross regional lymph node metastases
N3 (C/H)	Extraregional lymph node metastases
NX	Minimal requirements have not been met
M: *Distant Metastases*†	
M0	No evidence of metastases
M1	Elevated acid phosphatase only (three consecutive elevations)
M2 (V/B)	Visceral (V) and/or bone (B) metastases
MX	Minimal requirements not met
* TBC, in addition to the TC categories, requires TB specification of the extent of the intracapsular cancer. † Includes lymph nodes.	
Abbreviations: TUR, transurethral resection.	

Additional Diagnostic Testing

Computed tomography (CT) scan of the pelvis may be used to evaluate the pelvic lymph nodes for possible metastatic spread.

Bone scans are also useful for ruling out metastatic disease. Bone scans are rarely positive unless the PSA value is greater than 10.

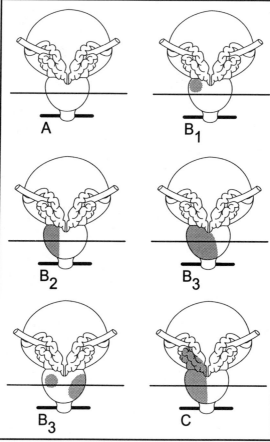

FIGURE 9.2 — FINDINGS ON DIGITAL RECTAL PALPATION

A

B_1

B_2

B_3

B_3

C

Approximated here are the palpable findings on digital rectal examination for clinical stages TA and TB1 through TB3 according to the Whitmore clinical staging system (see Table 9.1)

Adapted from Stamey TA, McNeal JE. Adenocarcinoma of the prostate. In: Walsh PC, Retik AB, Stamey TA, eds. *Campbell's Urology*. Volume 2. Philadelphia, Pa: WB Saunders Co; 1992:1159-1221.

10 Treatment

Prostate cancer is an unusual malignancy because of its high prevalence and unpredictable course. In suggesting appropriate therapy, the surgeon must consider the patient's age and medical condition and the stage of the tumor.

Radical Prostatectomy

For patients with cancer confined to the prostate who are no older than age 70 and who have no major medical contraindication, most urologic surgeons favor radical prostatectomy. This procedure involves:
- Pelvic lymphadenectomy for staging
- Resection of entire prostate, prostatic capsule, and seminal vesicles: potency is dependent on preservation of nerves outside of capsule
- Anastomosis of bladder neck to urethral stump; continence depends on preservation of urethral external sphincter.

Complications of radical prostatectomy include:
- Blood loss
- Incontinence
- Impotence
- Rectal injury
- Deep venous thrombosis (DVT)
- Bladder neck contracture.

Recent advances in this procedure include:
- Autologous blood donation, which minimizes risk of transfusion

- Nerve-sparing surgical technique with emphasis on identification and preservation of nerves required for potency
- Surgical techniques that result in less blood loss and preservation of the external sphincter
- Use of pneumatic compression boots to increase venous return, decrease DVT.

External Beam Radiation

Radiation was developed as a primary treatment in prostatic carcinoma because of a desire to avoid the impotence and occasional incontinence associated with radical prostatectomy. In most series, dosages of 7000 cGY are administered to the prostate and 5000 cGY to the lymph nodes over 6 weeks.

The results of radiation therapy are difficult to evaluate because:
- PSA levels usually go down, but repeat prostate biopsy often is positive
- Staging of the tumor is difficult without lymphadenectomy
- Radiation doses and targeting are operator-dependent.

Overall (not disease-free) 5-, 10-, and 15-year survival rates are comparable to those associated with radical prostatectomy. Complications include:
- Gastrointestinal (GI) tract problems (diarrhea, rectal pain, tenesmus)
- Urinary frequency
- Dysuria
- Urethral stricture
- Erectile dysfunction.

External beam therapy has recently been used for patients who have recurrent localized disease at the urethro-vesical junction after radical prostatectomy.

Serum PSA may be used to monitor the efficacy of therapy in this setting.

Radioactive Implantation

The placement of iodine-125 (^{125}I) or radioactive paladium seeds directly into the prostate theoretically delivers a high dose of radioactivity closer to the lesion. Initial trials showed no advantage over other treatment modalities, but more recently, sonography and computed tomography (CT) scan have provided better visualization of the prostate and several investigators are currently repeating the implantation technique with radiologic guidance. Long-term (5, 10 and 15 years) follow-ups will be necessary to assess the success rate, however, so the technique is still experimental.

Cryosurgery

In this relatively new alternative to the management of localized prostate cancer, the prostate is approached transperineally with two or more cryoprobes (serially or simultaneously) under transrectal ultrasound (US) guidance, and the tumor is frozen. This procedure remains investigational and long-term follow-up has not yet been reported.

Preliminary results suggest the procedure may be an effective alternative treatment for localized prostate cancer with minimal associated morbidity.

Hormone Ablation Therapy

Once prostatic cancer invades through the prostatic capsule or metastasizes, surgery or local noninvasive intervention is not effective in limiting the disease. At this point, hormonal ablation therapy should be considered, given testosterone's active stimulation of prostate cancer cell growth. Since 95% of testosterone is produced by the testis, the simplest, most direct way to produce androgen deprivation is bilateral orchiectomy. The other 5% of testosterone is contributed by the adrenal androgens dehydro-3-epiandrosterone and androstenedione. Thus, complete ablation of androgen sources would require either adrenalectomy or blockade of the effect of adrenal as well as testicular testosterone.

In very advanced disease – associated with impending spinal cord compression or bilateral hydronephrosis, for example – bilateral orchiectomy is the treatment of choice. Otherwise metastatic disease can be treated equally effectively with surgery and medical therapies (Table 10.1).

Androgen deprivation can be attained by three pharmaceutical approaches as well as by orchiectomy (Figure 10.1):

- Administration of exogenous estrogens such as diethylstilbestrol (DES)
- Use of analogues of luteinizing hormone-releasing hormone (LHRH), which inhibit the release of pituitary gonadotropins
- Combined androgen blockade using LHRH agonists plus antiandrogens that block androgens at target tissues.

The adrenal suppressing drug aminoglutethimide (indicated for Cushing's syndrome) and the antifungal agent ketoconazole, both of which block a variety of steroid biosynthetic pathways, have also been used with some efficacy in patients with advanced cancer.

Androgen deprivation produces subjective improvement in about 80% of patients and objective evidence of tumor regression in nearly 50%.

TABLE 10.1 — ANDROGEN ABLATION FOR PROSTATIC CANCER

Level	Agent	Sequelae	Dose
Pituitary, hypothalamus	Estrogens	Gynecomastia, hot flashes, thromboembolic disease, impotence	1 to 3 mg daily
	LHRH agonists	Impotence, hot flashes, gynecomastia, rarely anemia	Monthly injection
Adrenal	Ketoconazole	Adrenal insufficiency, nausea, gynecomastia, hepatic toxicity	400 mg 3 times daily
	Aminoglutethimide	Adrenal insufficiency, nausea, rash, ataxia	250 mg 4 times daily
	Glucocorticoids	Gastrointestinal bleeding, fluid retention	Prednisone: 20 to 40 mg daily
Testis	Orchiectomy	Gynecomastia, hot flashes, impotence	—
Prostate cell	Antiandrogens	No impotence when used alone; nausea, diarrhea	Flutamide: 250 mg 3 times daily

Abbreviations: LHRH, luteinizing hormone-releasing hormone.

10

FIGURE 10.1 — PROSTATIC CANCER DRUG THERAPY: SITES OF ACTION

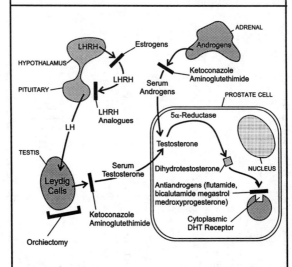

A number of approaches to androgen deprivation are currently available. Estrogens, in inhibiting the release of luteinizing hormone-releasing hormone (LHRH) from the hypothalamus, reduce the release of luteinizing hormone (LH) from the anterior pituitary, thus diminishing stimulation of the testes to produce testosterone. The LHRH analogues stimulate, then down-regulate the release of LH from the anterior pituitary. The testes, which produce most of the testosterone, can be removed by orchiectomy. Ketoconazole and aminoglutethimide inhibit testosterone directly in the testes and indirectly in the adrenal glands. In the prostate cell, testosterone is converted into dihydrotestosterone (DHT) by the enzyme 5α-reductase. True antiandrogens such as flutamide, bicalutamide, and certain progestational agents produce complete androgen blockade by preventing the binding of DHT to its cytoplasmic receptor.

■ Estrogens

Estrogen indirectly inhibits testosterone synthesis by inhibiting the release of LHRH and, in turn, of luteinizing hormone (LH), which acts at the Leydig cells in the testes to control testosterone production. Estrogens used in the treatment of advanced prostate cancer include:

- Diethylstilbestrol (DES), 1 to 2 mg/day
- Premarin, 1 to 10 mg/day
- Ethinyl estradiol, 0.5 to 1.0 mg/day.

The side effects of estrogen therapy include:

- Fluid retention
- Gynecomastia
- Impotence
- Increased incidence of deep venous thrombosis and other thromboembolic complications (DES).

■ LHRH Analogues

Short-term administration of these agents produces surges in follicle-stimulating hormone (FSH) and LH levels and, in turn, a "flare" in testosterone release. After 1 to 2 weeks, however, testosterone levels are reduced, presumably as a result of a decreased number of LHRH receptors in the pituitary, caused by overstimulation of LHRH down-regulation. At this point, there is a concomitant fall in testosterone and dihydrotestosterone levels. The currently available LHRH agonists are:

- Leuprolide acetate, 7.5 mg, IM, q 28 days; 22.5 mg, IM, q 3 months
- Goserelin acetate, 3.6 mg, SC, q 28 days; 10.8 mg, SC, q 3 months.

The initial flare may cause increased bone pain in the first week of therapy as well as a rise in PSA levels. The flare reaction can be greatly blunted by starting the nonsteroidal antiandrogen flutamide (see below) simultaneously or by 1 day of therapy with ketoconazole.

LHRH agonists should be avoided in any patients with metastatic cancer who has any suggestion of neurologic symptoms since a potential for spinal cord injury exists in the presence of vertebral metastases.

Adverse Reactions

In 8% or more of patients, leuprolide and goserelin were associated with adverse reactions, including:

- Leuprolide (Lupron)
  - General pain
  - Injection site reaction
  - Hot flashes/sweats
  - Gastrointestinal disorders
  - Joint disorders
  - Insomnia/sleep disorders
  - Neuromuscular disorders
  - Skin reaction
  - Testicular atrophy
  - Urinary disorders
- Goserelin (Zoladex)
  - Hot flashes
  - Sexual dysfunction
  - Decreased erections
  - Lower urinary tract symptoms
  - Lethargy
  - Pain (worsened in first 30 days).

■ Antiandrogens

Although bilateral orchiectomy, estrogens, and LHRH agonists eliminate or markedly suppress androgen production by the testes, the weakly androgenic steroids from the adrenal cortex remain and are converted into strong androgens in the peripheral tissues, including the prostate. Progestational agents suppress the pituitary's release of LHRH and also block the binding of dihydrotestosterone (DHT) to cytoplasmic receptors in prostate cells. The available agents (indicated for breast and endometrial cancer) are:

- Megestrol acetate, 120 mg/day
- Medroxyprogesterone acetate, 20 to 200 mg/day.

A major disadvantage of the progestational agents is their short-term effectiveness; testosterone levels begin to rise within a few days of treatment. The drugs' major adverse effect is impotence.

The more effective and now more commonly used nonsteroidal antiandrogens act solely as competitive inhibitors for DHT and testosterone receptors in the prostate. Two formulations are currently available:

- Flutamide, 250 mg, q8hrs
- Bicalutamide, 50 mg daily.

Both nonsteroidal antiandrogen agents are administered in combination with an LHRH analogue to achieve complete androgen source ablation.

Adverse Reactions

In a multicenter, double-blind, controlled trial comparing flutamide and bicalutamide, each in combination with an LHRH analogue, a number of adverse cardiovascular, digestive, and urogenital adverse events were documented (see Table 10.2).

■ Aminoglutethimide

Aminoglutethimide (750 to 2000 mg/day) inhibits adrenocortical steroid synthesis by blocking conversion of cholesterol to Δ^5-pregnenolone, resulting in decreased production of adrenal glucocorticoids, mineralocorticoids, estrogens, and androgens. A compensatory increase in adrenocorticotropic hormone (ACTH) requires simultaneous administration of hydrocortisone.

TABLE 10.2 — ADVERSE EXPERIENCE WITH FLUTAMIDE AND BICALUTAMIDE, EACH IN COMBINATION WITH LHRH ANALOGUE

Reaction	Flutamide	Bicalutamide
Hot flashes	50%	49%
Constipation	12%	17%
Nausea	11%	11%
Diarrhea	24%	10%
Liver enzyme increase*	10%	6%
Nocturia	11%	9%
Hematuria	5%	7%
Urinary tract infection	6%	6%
Impotence	7%	5%
Gynecomastia	6%	5%
Urinary incontinence	5%	2%

* AST, ALT or both. Periodic liver function tests should be considered.

Abbreviations: LHRH, luteinizing hormone-releasing hormone; AST, aspartate aminotransferase; ALT, alanine aminotransferase.

Adverse reactions to aminoglutethimide therapy include:

- Anorexia
- Nausea
- Skin rash
- Lethargy
- Vertigo
- Nystagmus
- Hypothyroidism.

■ **Ketoconazole**

This antifungal drug (400 mg q8hrs) impairs the production of androgen by inhibiting the enzymes of gonadal and adrenal corticosteroid synthesis. Castration levels of androgens occur within 4 to 8 hours of a 400 mg oral dose of ketoconazole. It is primarily helpful when there is a need for a rapid androgen response, such as occurs in impending spinal cord compression. Among ketoconazole's disadvantages are the frequent daily doses and the fact that breakthrough occurs after 1 month's treatment.

Adverse reactions to ketoconazole include:
- Weakness
- Lethargy
- Hepatic dysfunction
- Impotence
- GI tract upset
- Gynecomastia.

Immediate versus Deferred Treatment

The controversy regarding whether to treat asymptomatic advanced prostatic cancer when diagnosed or to wait until an indication of progression occurs has been addressed by a number of investigators over more than 2 decades. A Veterans Administration Cooperative Research Group study published in 1976 concluded that treatment can be delayed. At least four later studies reported significant differences in favor of early hormonal therapy in patients with radical prostatectomies who are found to have pelvic node metastases.

Early hormonal ablation, however, may select for hormone-resistant cancer cells. Long-term, randomized studies are necessary to resolve this controversy.

Hormone Refractory Disease

Although 75% of patients respond to androgen blockade, hormone refractory disease appears after a median of 18 months of endocrine manipulation and is attributed to the selection and/or cloning of preexisting or de novo appearing hormone-independent or resistant cell lines. A number of chemotherapeutic protocols have been developed using such agents as cisplatin, Adriamycin, cyclophosphamide, fluorouracil, lemustine, decarbazine, and methotrexate. However, only 10% of patient have had favorable responses to the therapy with short remissions usually lasting for less than 6 months.

In vitro studies have demonstrated the efficacy of the growth-factor inhibitor suramin in reducing cellular proliferation of androgen-dependent prostate-cancer cells. Initial clinical trials using high-dose suramin as monotherapy in patients with hormone-resistant disease have shown some promise but duration of response has been short lived and suramin toxicity is a problem.

Palliative treatment of late-stage metastatic prostate cancer includes:

- Steroids, ketoconazole, or IV stilbestrol for spinal cord compression (or emergency decompression laminectomy)
- Radiotherapy of metastatic sites causing pain (35% to 42% of patients experience pain relief).

PART 5

CASE HISTORIES AND SELECTED READINGS

11   Case Histories

The following case presentations are designed to demonstrate some of the treatment options available to patients with the four prostatitis syndromes, benign prostatic hyperplasia, and prostatic cancer.

Prostatitis

(Figure 11.1)

■ Case 1

A 60-year-old diabetic man presents to his primary-care physician with complaints of dysuria, decreasing force of urinary stream, fever, and chills of 2 days duration. On physical examination, he has a temperature of 102° F but no flank pain. His testes are soft and nontender without evidence of epididymitis. On rectal examination, the prostate is extremely tender, hot, and boggy without localized fluctuance.

This patient has acute prostatitis and should be hospitalized. Blood and urine cultures, complete blood count (CBC), and Sequential Multiple Analysis (SMA-6) + creatinine should be ordered before starting broad-spectrum intravenous antibiotics (ampicillin plus gentamicin). Microscopic examination of the urine and gram stain are also indicated. The patient should be monitored for progressive sepsis. His voiding should also be monitored, and if significant urinary retention is present, a suprapubic tube should be placed by the urologist. No urethral instrumentation (ie, Foley catheter) should be performed during acute prostatitis. Once the test results are returned, the drug may be changed to a specific antibiotic that treats the urinary infection.

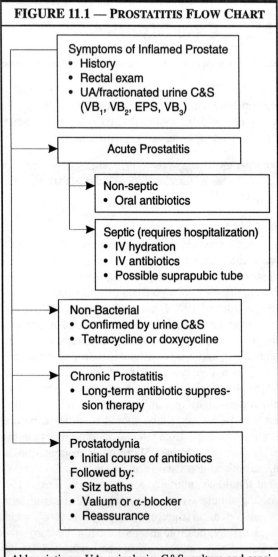

FIGURE 11.1 — PROSTATITIS FLOW CHART

Symptoms of Inflamed Prostate
- History
- Rectal exam
- UA/fractionated urine C&S
  (VB_1, VB_2, EPS, VB_3)

Acute Prostatitis

Non-septic
- Oral antibiotics

Septic (requires hospitalization)
- IV hydration
- IV antibiotics
- Possible suprapubic tube

Non-Bacterial
- Confirmed by urine C&S
- Tetracycline or doxycycline

Chronic Prostatitis
- Long-term antibiotic suppression therapy

Prostatodynia
- Initial course of antibiotics
Followed by:
- Sitz baths
- Valium or α-blocker
- Reassurance

Abbreviations: UA, urinalysis; C&S, culture and sensitivity testing; VB, voided bladder; EPS, expressed prostatic secretions; IV, intravenous.

■ Case 2

A sexually active, 35-year-old man complains of urinary frequency, dysuria, and vague perineal pain. He denies past urologic problems. Scrotal examination is normal and there is no evidence of epididymitis and no urethral discharge.

Before performing the rectal examination, the physician should consider the diagnosis of prostatitis and initiate sequential urine analysis. The patient may be started on a broad-spectrum antibiotic such as TMP-SMX, bid, until culture results are returned.

> **Note**: If urethral discharge is noted prior to the examination, and gonorrhea or chlamydia urethritis is suspected, the patient should be given an intramuscular injection of ceftriaxone sodium, 250 mg, and either tetracycline, 500 mg qid, or doxycycline, 100 mg bid, for 7 days.

■ Case 3

A 39-year-old man presents with a dull ache in his rectum. He states that he has had similar episodes in the past and has been treated with TMP-SMX, ciprofloxacin, carbenicillin, and tetracycline with variable results. He feels he needs "more antibiotics."

This patient's history is typical for prostatodynia. However, he should be carefully evaluated to rule out other prostate disease. Physical examination should look for hemorrhoids as well as for prostate tenderness induration or nodules. Appropriate urine and expressed prostatic secretion (EPS) samples should be taken. The patient may be prescribed a course of antibiotics, such as tetracycline, 500 mg qid, for 10 days. If on his return visit all cultures are negative and prostatodynia is still suspected, he may be prescribed sitz baths and possibly an α-blocker or low-dose diazepam.

■ Case 4

A 59-year-old patient presents with urinary frequency, dysuria, and occasional decreased force of urinary stream. He states that he was treated with antibiotics for prostatitis approximately 2 years ago and has had two urinary tract infections during the past 8 months. On rectal examination, he has a moderately tender prostate without fluctuance or calculi.

This patient has symptoms of chronic prostatitis. The physician should order urine culture and sensitivity testing (C&S) and EPS culture and start the patient on a broad-spectrum antibiotic such as TMP-SMX or ciprofloxacin. Chronic infection may require 2 or 3 weeks to be completely eradicated. Alternatively, the patient may have a nidus of infection such as a prostatic calculus, which may require long-term antibiotic therapy or even transurethral resection.

Benign Prostatic Hyperplasia

(Figure 11.2)

■ Case 1

A 63-year-old patient presents with complaints of frequency of urination and nocturia once per night. He denies having dysuria, states that he voids with an adequate force of stream and feels that he empties his bladder adequately.

This is the typical presentation of a patient with early prostatism and an unstable bladder. Diagnostic testing should include prostate-specific antigen (PSA) level, urine C&S, and a thorough genital and rectal examination to evaluate the size of the prostate and any irregularities. The patient should be advised to decrease caffeine, alcohol, and fluid intake before bedtime. Symptoms should be evaluated on follow-up visits, and if they progress, the patient should be started on medical treatment such as an α-adrenergic blocker or finasteride.

114

FIGURE 11.2 — BENIGN PROSTATIC HYPERPLASIA FLOW CHART

Symptom Assessment:
- History
- Physical exam (rectal)
- UA, urine C&S, PSA, PAP, BUN/creatinine

Mild:
- Observe minor lifestyle changes

Moderate:
- Observation
  OR
- Drug therapy

Severe:
- TUIP
- TURP (Gold Standard)
- Open prostatectomy

Poor Surgical Risk:
- Prostatic stent
- TUIP

New Procedures:
- Microwave hyperthermia
- Laser ablation

Abbreviations: UA, urinalysis; C&S, culture and sensitivity testing; PSA, prostate-specific antigen; PAP, prostatic acid phosphatase; BUN, blood urea nitrogen; TUIP, transurethral incision of the prostate; TURP, transurethral resection of the prostate.

■ Case 2

A 69-year-old patient presents with decreased force of stream, frequency, and nocturia. He says he has had mild symptoms for several years, but lately he has to "really strain to empty his bladder." He also has significant medical problems, including asthma, congestive heart failure, and hypertension, and he had a myocardial infarction 2 years ago.

This patient has significant symptoms of prostatism that seem to be progressing. After physical examination and urine and serum studies are performed, he should be informed of his options. Although a transurethral resection of the prostate (TURP) would probably relieve his symptoms, his medical condition puts him at increased risk for surgery. He can be offered a trial of drug treatment, such as an α-adrenergic blocker or finasteride, or a less invasive procedure such as microwave therapy or transurethral incision of the prostate (TUIP).

■ Case 3

A 72-year-old patient complains of decreased force of stream, nocturia, and two episodes of urinary retention. On rectal examination, he has a markedly enlarged prostate without induration, nodules, or tenderness. His urine C&S has been negative and his PSA is 3.8. The patient has tried an α-adrenergic agent but did not take it regularly.

This patient has progressive symptoms of prostatism. Although he could be prescribed another trial of drug therapy or minimally invasive therapy (such as microwave therapy), his markedly enlarged prostate probably warrants TURP.

Note: Patients should be informed that once they start on drug therapy, they must continue to take their medication indefinitely as prescribed or the symptoms may recur.

Case 4

An 84-year-old, bedridden nursing home patient with chronic obstructive pulmonary disease and Alzheimer's disease is unable to void. He has been treated with an indwelling catheter but the nursing home staff are concerned about potential urinary tract infections.

Chronic indwelling catheters will cause colonization of the bladder with bacteria, increasing the risk of epididymitis, prostatitis, and subsequent urosepsis. This patient should undergo urodynamic testing to confirm that his bladder has normal compliance. Because of his poor medical condition, a minimally invasive procedure, such as placement of a prostatic stent or TUIP, should be performed.

Prostate Cancer

(Figure 11.3)

Case 1

A 53-year-old patient states that he had an elevated PSA of 6.0 drawn as part of a routine physical examination. He has no significant medical problems and voids normally. His rectal examination is normal.

An increasing number of men are undergoing such routine PSA testing. This patient should have a repeat PSA test and a rectal examination by a urologist. If the PSA level is persistently elevated with a normal rectal examination, he should be examined with rectal sonography and random transrectal biopsies should be taken. Positive biopsies call for a metastatic workup: prostatic acid phosphatase (PAP), alkaline phosphatase (ALP), and bone scan. In the absence of metastases, the patient should be informed of his therapeutic options: radical prostatectomy, external beam radiation, or observation. Because of his age and good medical condition, a radical prostatec-

11

FIGURE 11.3 — PROSTATE CANCER FLOW CHART

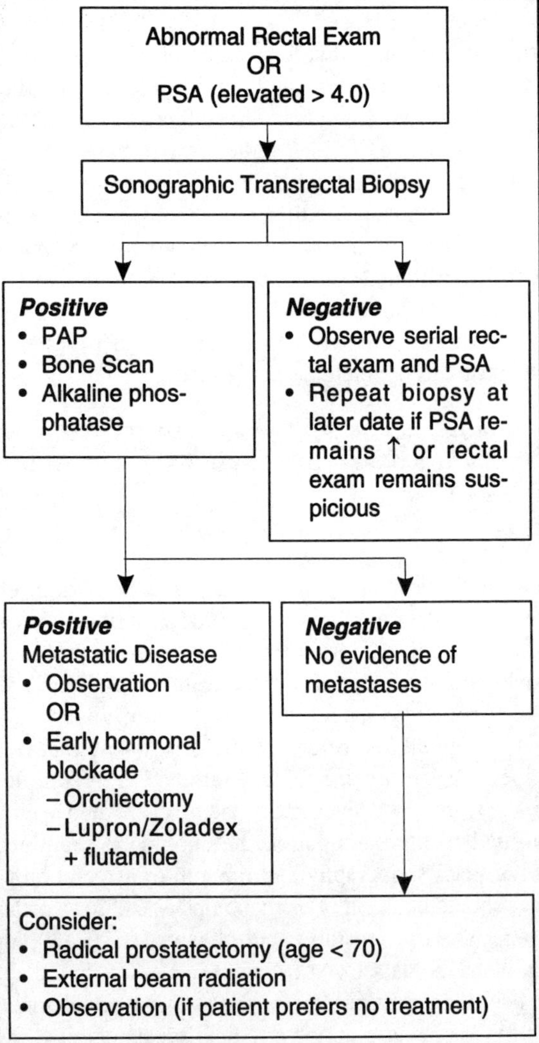

Abnormal Rectal Exam
OR
PSA (elevated > 4.0)

↓

Sonographic Transrectal Biopsy

Positive
- PAP
- Bone Scan
- Alkaline phosphatase

Negative
- Observe serial rectal exam and PSA
- Repeat biopsy at later date if PSA remains ↑ or rectal exam remains suspicious

Positive
Metastatic Disease
- Observation OR
- Early hormonal blockade
  - Orchiectomy
  - Lupron/Zoladex + flutamide

Negative
No evidence of metastases

Consider:
- Radical prostatectomy (age < 70)
- External beam radiation
- Observation (if patient prefers no treatment)

Abbreviations: PSA, prostate-specific antigen; PAP, prostatic acid phosphatase.

tomy is suggested. If the biopsies are negative, on the other hand, the patient should have a repeat PSA in 3 months, and if it remains elevated or continues to rise, repeat biopsies should be performed.

■ Case 2

A 66-year-old patient presents with a discrete prostatic nodule diagnosed by his internist. His PSA is 11, and he is otherwise healthy.

This patient should undergo repeat rectal examinations by the urologist to confirm that the lesion is indeed confined to the prostate (stage B). Diagnostic testing should include ultrasound-guided transrectal biopsy as well as PAP, ALP, and bone scan. If the tumor is confined to the prostate, he should be offered a choice of radical prostatectomy, external beam radiation, or observation.

■ Case 3

A 76-year-old in good health presents with a PSA level of 36. His rectal examination reveals a large prostatic lesion fixed to the pelvic side wall (stage C). Prostate biopsy is positive for cancer. He voids without problems.

The patient should be tested for PAP and ALP levels and should have a bone scan for staging purposes. Because of his age and the stage of the tumor he is not a candidate for radical prostatectomy. If there is no indication of metastatic disease, he should be offered external beam radiation for local disease control or observation. Hormonal ablation may be delayed until further metastatic spread occurs.

■ Case 4

An 82-year-old patient presents with right hip pain. He has a history of hypertension and is a smoker. His PSA level is 130 and PAP is 8.0. Rectal examination reveals a firm, nodular prostate.

This patient probably has metastatic prostate cancer. He should have a transrectal biopsy and bone scan. Hormonal blockade, consisting of castration or combination treatment with a luteinizing hormone-releasing hormone (LHRH) agonist (leuprolide or goserelin) plus an antiandrogen agent should be started as soon as possible.

> **Note**: Unless given simultaneously with an antiandrogen, the LHRH agonist may cause an initial "flare," defined as a worsening of symptoms before testosterone levels eventually fall. Once medical castration is initiated it must be continued for the patient's lifetime. If a patient presents with symptoms of spinal cord compression (severe back pain, paraesthesia or paralysis), emergency hospitalization is necessary. Such patients require spinal x-ray or computed tomography (CT) scan and emergency neurology consultation. They are usually started on IV steroids and ketoconazole to lower the testosterone. Emergency orchiectomy is also an option. LHRH agonists would not be a good option because it takes several weeks for them to lower testosterone and relieve symptoms.

12 Selected Readings

Prostatitis

Childs SJ. Current concepts in the treatment of urinary tract infections and prostatitis. *Am J Med.* 1991;91(suppl 6A):120S-123S.

Cunha BA, Marx J, Gingrich D. Managing prostatitis in the elderly. *Geriatrics.* 1991;46:60-63.

Fowler JE. Prostatitis. In: Gillenwater J, Grayhack JT, Howards S, et al, eds. *Adult and Pediatric Urology.* Volume 2. St. Louis, Mo: Mosby Yearbook; 1991:1395-1423.

Fowler JE. Bacteriuria and associated infections of the reproductive system in men. In: *Urinary Tract Infection and Inflammation.* Chicago, Ill: Yearbook Medical Publishers, Inc; 1989:92-123.

Lowentritt JE, Kawahara K, Human LG, Hellstrom WJ, Domingue GJ. Bacterial infection in prostatodynia. *J Urol.* 1995;154:1378-1381.

Meares EM Jr. Prostatitis and related disorders. In: Walsh PC, Retik AB, Stamey TA, eds. *Campbell's Urology.* Volume 1. Philadelphia, Pa: WB Saunders Co; 1992:807-822.

Miller JL, Rothman I, Bavendam TG, Berger RE. Prostatodynia and interstitial cystitis: one and the same? *Urology.* 1995;45:587-590.

Moul JW. Prostatitis: Sorting out the different causes. *Postgrad Med.* 1993;94:191-194.

Presti JC Jr, Stoller M, Carroll PR. Urology. In: Tierney LM, McPhee SF, Papadakis MA, eds. *Current Medical Diagnosis and Treatment.* Stamford, Conn: Appleton & Lange; 1996:830-833.

Rubin RH. Infections of the urinary tract. In: Rubenstein E, Federman DD, eds. *Scientific American Medicine.* New York, NY: Scientific American, Inc; 1996:1-11.

Terasaki T, Watanabe H, Saitoh M, Uchida M, Okamura S, Shimizu K. Magnetic resonance angiography in prostatodynia. *Eur Urol.* 1995;27:280-285.

Benign Prostatic Hyperplasia

Ahmed M, Bell T, Lawrence WT, Ward JP, Watson GM. Transurethral microwave thermotherapy (Prostatron version 2.5) compared with transurethral resection of the prostate for the treatment of benign prostatic hyperplasia: a randomized, controlled, parallel study. *Br J Urol.* 1997;79:181-185.

Boyle P, Gould AL, Roehrborn CG. Prostate volume predicts outcome of treatment of benign prostatic hyperplasia with finasteride: meta-analysis of randomized clinical trials. *Urology.* 1996;48:398-405.

Chapple CR, Wyndaele JJ, Nordling J, Boeminghaus F, Ypma AF, Abrams P. Tamsulosin, the first prostate-selective α_{1A}-adrenoceptor antagonist: a meta-analysis of two randomized, placebo-controlled, multicentre studies in patients with benign prostatic obstruction (symptomatic BPH). *Eur Urol.* 1996;29:155-167.

Chapple CR. Selective alpha 1-adrenoceptor antagonists in benign prostatic hyperplasia: rationale and clinical experience. *Eur Urol.* 1996;29:129-144.

Chiou RK, Chen WS, Akbari A, Foley S, Lynch B, Taylor RJ. Long-term outcome of prostatic stent treatment for benign prostatic hyperplasia. *Urology.* 1996;48:589-593.

Elhilali MM, Ramsey EW, Barkin J, et al. A multicenter, randomized, double-blind, placebo-controlled study to evaluate the safety and efficacy of terazosin in the treatment of benign prostatic hyperplasia. *Urology.* 1996;47:335-342.

Gerber GS, Kim JH, Contreras BA, Steinberg GD, Rukstalis DB. An observational urodynamic evaluation of men with lower urinary tract symptoms treated with doxazosin. *Urology.* 1996;47:840-844.

Girman CJ, Kolman C, Liss CL, Bolognese JA, Binkowitz BS, Stoner E. Effects of finasteride on health-related quality of life in men with symptomatic benign prostatic hyperplasia. Finasteride Study Group. *Prostate.* 1996;29:83-90.

Kabalin JN, Bite G, Doll S. Neodymium:YAG laser coagulation prostatectomy: 3 years of experience with 227 patients. *J Urol.* 1996;155:181-185.

Kaplan SA, Meade-D'Alisera P, Quiñones S, Soldo KA. Doxazosin in physiologically and pharmacologically normotensive men with benign prostatic hyperplasia. *Urology.* 1995;46:512-517.

Kawabe K. Efficacy and safety of tamsulosin in the treatment of benign prostatic hyperplasia. *Br J Urol.*1995;76(suppl 1):63-67.

Klus GT, Nakamura J, Li JS, et al. Growth inhibition of human prostate cells *in vitro* by novel inhibitors of androgen synthesis. *Cancer Res.* 1996;56:4956-4964.

Lepor H, Williford WO, Barry MJ, et al. The efficacy of terazosin, finasteride, or both in benign prostatic hyperplasia. *N Engl J Med.* 1996;335:533-539.

Moore E, Bracken B, Bremner W, et al. Proscar: five-year experience. *Eur Urol.* 1995;28:304-309.

Narayan P, Trachtenberg J, Lepor H, et al. A dose-response study of the effect of flutamide on benign prostatic hyperplasia: results of a multicenter study. *Urology.* 1996;47:497-504.

Oesterling JE. Benign prostatic hyperplasia. Medical and minimally invasive treatment options. *N Engl J Med.* 1995;332:99-109.

Pool JL. Doxazosin: a new approach to hypertension and benign prostatic hyperplasia. *Br J Clin Pract.* 1996;50:154-163.

Ricciotti G, Bozzo W, Perachino M, Pezzica C, Puppo P. Heat-expansible permanent intraurethral stents for benign prostatic hyperplasia and urethral strictures. *J Endourol.* 1995;9:417-422.

Rittmaster RS. Finasteride. *N Engl J Med.* 1994;330:120-125.

Roehrborn CG, Siegel RL. Safety and efficacy of doxazosin in benign prostatic hyperplasia: a pooled analysis of three double-blind, placebo-controlled studies. *Urology.* 1996;48:406-415.

Roehrborn CG, Oesterling JE, Auerbach S, et al. The Hytrin Community Assessment Trial study: a one-year study of terazosin versus placebo in the treatment of men with symptomatic benign prostatic hyperplasia. HYCAT Investigator Group. *Urology.* 1996;47:159-168.

Schulman CC, Cortvriend J, Jonas U. Tamsulosin, the first prostate-selective α_{1A}-adrenoceptor antagonist. Analysis of a multinational, multicentre, open-label study assessing the long-term efficacy and safety in patients with benign prostatic obstruction (symptomatic BPH). European Tamsulosin Study Group. *Eur Urol.* 1996;29:145-154.

Soeishi Y, Matsushima H, Watanabe T, Higuchi S, Cornelisson K, Ward J. Absorption, metabolism and excretion of tamsulosin hydrochloride in man. *Xenobiotica.* 1996;26:637-645.

Steiner JF. Clinical pharmacokinetics and pharmacodynamics of finasteride. *Clin Pharmacokinet.* 1996;30:16-27.

Sullivan LD, McLoughlin ME, Goldenberg LG, Gleave ME, Marich KW. Early experience with high-intensity focused ultrasound for the treatment of benign prostatic hypertrophy. *J Urol.* 1997;79:172-176.

Thomas KJ, Cornaby AJ, Hammadeh M, Philp T, Matthews PN. Transurethral vaporization of the prostate: a promising new technique. *Br J Urol.* 1997;79:186-189.

Walsh PC. Treatment of benign prostatic hyperplasia. *N Engl J Med.* 1996;335:586-587. Editorial.

Walsh PC. Benign prostatic hyperplasia. In: Walsh PC, Retik AB, Stamey TA, eds. *Campbell's Urology.* Volume 1. Philadelphia, Pa: WB Saunders Co; 1992:1009-1027.

Prostate Cancer

Bologna M, Muzi P, Biordi L, Festuccia C, Vincentini C. Finasteride dose-dependently reduces the proliferation rate of the LnCap human prostatic cancer cell line *in vitro. Urology.* 1995;45:282-290.

Edelstein RA, Babayan RK. Managing prostate cancer, Part I: localized disease. *Hosp Pract.* 1993;28:61-78.

Fornara P, Jocham D. Clinical study results of the new formulation leuprorelin acetate three-month depot for the treatment of advanced prostate carcinoma. *Urol Int.* 1996;56(suppl 1):18-22.

Garnick MB. Prostate cancer. In: Rubenstein E, Federman DD, eds. *Scientific American Medicine.* New York, NY: Scientific American, Inc; 1996:1-11.

Ford LG, Brawley OW, Perlman JA, Nayfield SG, Johnson KA, Kramer BS. The potential for hormonal prevention trials. *Cancer.* 1994;74(suppl 9):2726-2733.

Kehinde EO, Terry TR, Mistry N, Horsburgh T, Sandhu DP, Bell PR. UK studies on suramin therapy in hormone resistant prostate cancer. *Cancer Surv.* 1995;23:217-229.

Kelly WK, Curley T, Leibretz C, Dnistrian A, Schwartz M, Scher HI. Prospective evaluation of hydrocortisone and suramin in patients with androgen-independent prostate cancer. *J Clin Oncol.* 1995;13:2208-2213.

Kienle E, Lubben G. Efficacy and safety of leuporelin acetate depot for prostate cancer. The German Leuprorelin Study Group. *Urol Int.* 1996;56(suppl 1):23-30.

Kolvenbag GJ, Blackledge GR. Worldwide activity and safety of bicalutamide: a summary review. *Urology.* 1996;47(suppl 1A):70-79.

Kreis W, Budman DR, Calabro A. Unique synergism or antagonism of combinations of chemotherapeutic and hormonal agents in human prostate cancer cell lines. *Br J Urol.* 1997;79:196-202.

Kurhanewicz J, Vigneron DB, Hricak H, et al. Prostate cancer: metabolic response to cryosurgery as detected with 3D H-1 MR spectroscopic imaging. *Radiology.* 1996;200:489-496.

Lee F, Bahn DK, McHugh TA, Onik GM, Lee FJ Jr. US-guided percutaneous cryoablation of prostate cancer. *Radiology.* 1994;192:769-776.

Mahler C, Denis LJ. Hormone refractory disease. *Semin Surg Oncol.* 1995;11:77-83.

Medical Research Council Prostate Cancer Working Party Investigators Group. Immediate versus deferred treatment for advanced prostatic cancer: initial results of the Medical Research Council trial. *Br J Urol.* 1997;79:235-246.

Onik GM, Cohen JK, Reyes GD, Rubinsky B, Chang Z, Baust J. Transrectal ultrasound-guided percutaneous radical cryosurgical ablation of the prostate. *Cancer.* 1993;72:1291-1299.

12

Schellhammer P, Sharifi R, Block N, et al. Maximal androgen blockade for patients with metastatic prostate cancer: outcome of a controlled trial of bicalutamide versus flutamide, each in combination with luteinizing hormone-releasing hormone analogue therapy. *Urology.* 1996;47(suppl 1A):54-60.

Stamey TA, McNeal JE. Adenocarcinoma of the prostate. In: Walsh PC, Retik AB, Stamey TA, eds. *Campbell's Urology.* Volume 2. Philadelphia, Pa: WB Saunders Co; 1992:1159-1221.

Yachia D, Aridogan IA. The use of a removable stent in patients with prostate cancer and obstruction. *J Urol.* 1996;155:1956-1958.

Note: Page numbers in *italics* indicate figures;
page numbers followed by t indicate tables.